Suprapubic Lithotomy: The High Operation For Stone, Epicystotomy, Hypogastric Lithotomy (the High Apparatus).

William Tod Helmuth

SUPRAPUBIC LITHOTOMY.

THE HIGH OPERATION FOR STONE—EPICYSTOTOMY—HYPOGASTRIC LITHOTOMY—(THE HIGH APPARATUS).

BY

WM. TOD HELMUTH, M.D.,

PROFESSOR OF SURGERY IN THE NEW YORK HOMŒOPATHIC MEDICAL COLLEGE, SURGEON TO
THE HOMŒOPATHIC HOSPITAL ON WARD'S ISLAND, AND TO THE
HAHNEMANN HOSPITAL, NEW YORK, ETC., ETC.

*ILLUSTRATED WITH EIGHT LITHOGRAPHIC PLATES AND
NUMEROUS ENGRAVINGS ON WOOD.*

BOERICKE & TAFEL:

NEW YORK,
145 GRAND ST.

PHILADELPHIA,
1011 ARCH ST.

1882.

EW

BIBLIOGRAPHY.

American Journal of the Medical Sciences. July, 1875; July, 1877; April, 1878.

American Journal of the Medical Sciences. April, 1881.

American Journal of the Medical Sciences. January, 1878.

American Journal of the Medical Sciences. April, 1880.

American Journal of the Medical Sciences. January, 1880.

American Journal of the Medical Sciences. January, 1879.

Medical Times. December 18th, 1880.

Landmarks, Medical and Surgical. By Luther Holden, F.R.C.S. London, 1876.

Gross, On the Urinary Organs. 3d Ed., Philadelphia, 1876.

Handbuch der Topographischen Anatomie. Hyrtl. Vol. ii. Wien; 1860.

Ranking's Half Yearly Abstract of the Medical Sciences. Vol. xii, 1850, pp. 130.

Cooper, Samuel, Surgical Dictionary. New York, 1854.

Velpeau, A.A.L.M., Operative Surgery. Vol. iii, p. 947, et seq.

Belmas, Traité de la Cystotomie sus-pubienne. Paris, 1827.

Heister, D. L., Institutiones Chirurgicæ. Tom. ii. Amstelædami, MDCCXXXIX.

Van Buren, W. H., & Isaacs. Operative Surgery. New York, 1857.

Coulson, Diseases of the Bladder. Philadelphia, 1838.

Coulson, Diseases of the Bladder. Revised Edition. New York, 1881.

Günther, G. B., Operationem am Becken. Leipzig und Heidelberg, 1860.

Günther, G. B., Der hohe Steinschnitt. Leipzig, 1851.

Dupuytren, G., Lithotomie, Thèse. Paris, 1812. Concours pour la chaire de médecine opératoire.

Philosophical Transactions. Vol. xii. London (1700–1722–23.)

Transactions of the Provincial Medical and Surgical Association, 1850.

Cheselden, W., A Treatise on the High Operation for Stone. With xvii copper-plates. London, 1723.

Cheselden, W., The Anatomy of the Human Body. London, 1778.

Carpue, J. C., F.R.C.S., History of the High Operation for Stone. London, 1819.

Baseilhac Paschal. Eloge Historique de Frère Côme, de la Taille Laterale et celle de l'hypogastrique ou Haut Appareil. Paris, 1804.

Côme Frère. Nouvelle méthode d'extraire la pierre de la vessie par dessus la pubis qui on nomme vulgairement le Haut Appareil dans l'un et l'autre sexe, sans le secours d'aucun fluide retenu ne force dans la vessie. Paris, 1779.

Humphreys, G. M., Trans. and Provincial Medical and Surgical Association. Vol. v, London, 1851.

Mémoires de l'Académie Royale de Médecine. Paris, 1840.

Gibson, William, Institutes and Practice of Surgery. Vol. ii, Phila., 1835.

London Lancet. Vol. ii, 1841.

London Lancet. Vol. ii, 1858.

London Lancet. Vol. ii, 1873.

St. Louis Medical and Surgical Journal. 1865.

Dictionnaire Encyclop. des Sciences Médicale. Paris, vol. xxv, 1880.

Medical and Surgical History of the War of the Rebellion. Part ii, vol. ii.

Medico-Chirurgical Review, Lithotomy and Lithotrity compared. By Thomas King, M.D., M.R.C.S. London, 1832.

Medical Record. New York, January 25th, 1879.

Sharp, Samuel, A Treatise on the Operations of Surgery. London, 1747.

Holmes, A Treatise on Surgery, its Principles and Practice. Phila., 1876.

Spence, James, F.R.C.S., Lectures on Surgery. Vol. ii, Edinburgh, 1871.

Pirrie, Wm., F.R.S.E., The Principles and Practice of Surgery. London, 1873.

Gross, Samuel D., A System of Surgery. Philadelphia, vol. ii, p. 894.

Bryant, Thomas, F.R.C.S., The Practice of Surgery. London, 1872.

Hamilton, F. H., Principles and Practice of Surgery. New York, 1872.

Erichsen, John, The Science and Art of Surgery. Philadelphia, 1860.

Erichsen, John E., The Science and Art of Surgery. New Edition, ii vols. Philadelphia, 1878.

Latta, James, A Practical System of Surgery. In three volumes. Vol. i, London and Edinburgh, 1795.

Roberts, John B., American Edition of Bryant's System of Surgery. Philadelphia, 1881.

Holmes, T., A System of Surgery. In five volumes. New York, 1871, vol. iv.

London Medical and Surgical Repertory. Vol. xii–xiii.

Kirby, Cases with Observations on Wry-neck, etc., Medico-Chirurgical Soc. Edinburgh, vol. ii.

London Medical Gazette. Vol. i–v.

Transactions Medico-Chirurgical Soc. Edinburgh, vol. ii.

Bulletin de Thérapeutique. Vol. xcii.

Canadian Journal of Medical Sciences. Toronto, No. 2, Nov., 1881.

Dictionnaire de Méd. et de Chirurgie. Paris, 1831.

South's Translation of Chelius's System of Surgery. Philadelphia, 1847.

Bancal, A. P., Lithotomie et Lithotripsie. Bordeaux, 1839.

Hildanus, Guil., Fab. Opera quæ extant omnia. Frankofurte ad Mænum. 1646.

Cross, John Green, A Treatise on the Formation, Constituents, and Extraction of Urinary Calculi. Prize Essay. London, 1835.

Archives de Médecine. Paris, vols. xvii, xix, xx, xxi, xxvii.

Anderson's Quarterly of the Medical Sciences. London, 1824–26, vol. iii.

Edinburgh Journal of the Medical Sciences. 1826–27, vol. iii.

Sabattier, R. B., De la Médecine Opératoire. Nouvelle Edition, par J. L. Samson et L. J. Bégin. Four volumes. Paris, 1832.

Le Courrier Médical. Paris, 1876.

Poulet, A., Foreign Bodies in the Bladder. Vol. ii, New York, 1880.

FRONTISPIECE
REGIONAL ANATOMY OF PARTS CONCERNED IN EPICYSTOTOMY.

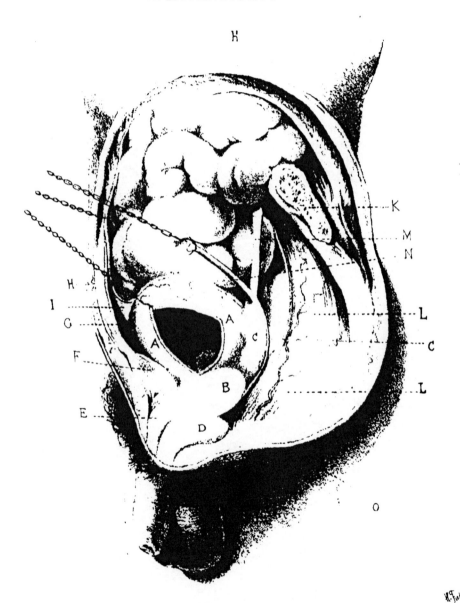

FRONTISPIECE.

Longitudinal Section of the Abdominal Cavity.

A. Bladder; portion of left wall removed.

B. Prostate gland.

C. Vesicula seminalis (left).

D. Bulb of urethra.

E. Crus penis.

F. Symphysis pubis.

G. Anterior wall of bladder, not covered by peritoneum.

H. Peritoneum reflected from fundus of bladder to abdominal wall.

I. Triangular space formed by the reflection of peritoneum, marking the site of the incision; generally covered with bladder fat.

K. Sacrum.

L. Rectum.

M. Ureter.

N. Vas deferens (left).

O. Anus.

PREFACE.

In these days, when the entire surgical world is so deeply interested in Bigelow's Litholapaxy,[*] or, as it should be named, "the American method of lithotrity," it would appear almost inappropriate to call attention to any form of lithotomy, especially to that one, which, in the estimation of many surgeons, is the most unreliable, and only to be performed under most peculiar circumstances. So convinced, however, is the author of these pages that epicystotomy will, before many years have passed, receive a high place among all the *cutting* operations for stone in the bladder, especially in those cases in which litholapaxy is inappropriate, that this essay is offered to the profession. The author, however, in this place, desires to give to Dr. C. W. Dulles, of Philadelphia, the credit of developing and prolonging an interest in epicystotomy, which otherwise would not have existed, and would state that it was from the perusal of his (Dr. Dulles) papers[†] that he was led to perform the operations which are herein detailed.

In the admiration, however, which is felt for the easy performance and comparative freedom from danger of the suprapubic method, the author would not be understood as considering it preferable to the crushing operation as it is performed to-day,[‡] for with the present appreciation of litholapaxy and its results,[§] perhaps if the second case recorded had been submitted to the lithotrite the patient might have recovered. The desire is simply to express the conviction that if a cutting operation be desirable, hypogastric lithotomy in many cases is preferable to all others, and to direct attention to the fact that a fair

---

[*] Lithotrity by a Single Operation. By Henry J. Bigelow, M.D. American Journal of the Medical Sciences. January, 1878, p. 117.

[†] Suprapubic Lithotomy. By C. W. Dulles, M.D. American Journal of the Medical Sciences. July, 1875; July, 1877; April, 1878.

[‡] *Vide* "Rapid Lithotrity with Evacuation." By E. L. Keyes, A.M., M.D. American Journal of the Medical Sciences. April, 1880.

[§] *Vide* "An Article on Litholapaxy." By R. F. Wier, M.D. American Journal of the Medical Sciences. January, 1880, p. 130.

estimate of it has not been arrived at by the majority of the profession, because, as a rule, only the most aggravated cases have been to it submitted.

Every candid surgeon of the present day, dispassionately considering the suprapubic method, compared with the various perineal and other operations for removing calculi from the bladder, must arrive at the conclusion that epi-cystotomy, from the anatomical construction of the parts incised, from its simplicity, and the advantage of *seeing* as well as *feeling* the varied steps of the operation, must often be the superior method. These views are gradually being entertained by the profession, as may be evinced by the newer methods of treating cystitis and enlarged prostate by an opening above the pubes after the manner of Sir Henry Thompson.*

When as much time and experience have been expended upon "the high operation" as have been given to lateral and median lithotomy, and *when an equal number of favorable cases have been submitted to it*, the results will be better than those furnished by any other cutting methods for the extraction of stone.

---

* Medical Times, December 18th, 1880.

CONTENTS

SUPRAPUBIC LITHOTOMY.

CHAPTER I.

A BRIEF HISTORY OF THE HIGH OPERATION.

In endeavoring to look into the remote history of suprapubic lithotomy, one is surprised to observe the many vicissitudes through which it has passed; sometimes standing high in the estimation of the profession, at other periods sinking entirely into oblivion. The history, however, is full of interest to those desiring to investigate the subject, for here and there throughout its literature, exhaustive monographs appear, exhibiting the zeal and perseverance of those, who from time to time have been the upholders of the operation.

In the whole history of hypogastric lithotomy, the most decidedly unique case in all its details is that of Jean de Dot, the smith, of Amsterdam, "who cut himself in the linea alba above the pubis, and took out of his bladder a stone as large as a hen's egg. The stone, the knife, and the portrait of the operator, may be seen to this day in the Museum at Leyden."[*]

Being anxious while investigating this subject to learn more of this remarkable case, I addressed a communication to Mr. Holden, inquiring if more details could be furnished. I received in a courteous reply, the following extract: "Jean de Dot, a smith of Amsterdam, cut a stone as big as a goose-egg out of his own bladder by the suprapubic operation; he used a pocket knife previously sharpened, and was assisted by his apprentices.

"This case happened in the seventeenth century, and the history is attested by the Burgomeister and Town Council, as also by the College of Surgeons."[†]

On a late visit to Holland, I took especial pains to visit the Anatomical Museum, at Leyden, and had the satisfaction of seeing the stone, the knife, which is an ordinary shoemaker's knife, not a pocket knife, as related by Hyrtl, and the certificate of the notary, "Pieter de Barry," with the date of "Maye, 1651." I observed also that the record reads Jean Doot, and not "de Dot," as is printed in several works of to-day.

---

[*] Landmarks, Medical and Surgical. By Luther Holden, F.R.C.S. London, J. Churchill, p. 31; also *vide* Gross on the Urinary Organs, 3d ed., Philadelphia, 1876, p. 293.

[†] Handbuch der Topographischen Anatomie, Hyrtl; vol. ii, p. 145; Wien, 1860.

It may be well here also to note the remarkable case of Josephi, in 1828, as recorded by Günther, in which a fœtus was removed by the high operation, having passed into the bladder, either from the Fallopian tube or ovary, and also another but more recent one, in which a stone was extracted at the umbilicus through an open urachus.*

The immense volume of some of the calculi which have been removed by the suprapubic method render the cases very remarkable.

Thus Vitellius extracted a calculus weighing ℥xxij, as related by Earle. The patient died. This case must have been among the earlier operations, as it is referred to by Hildanus, as quoted by Dulles. In Earle's paper, which was read on March 28th, 1820, the suprapubic method is not specified. It is also mentioned that Deguise, took from a patient, aged sixty-five years, a stone weighing ℥xxxj, which had been fruitlessly attempted through the perinæum. The patient died on the sixth day.

Uytterhœven cut out a concretion weighing two pounds, as quoted by Erichsen, Dulles, and others.

In Krimer's case the stone weighed ℥xxiij, the patient was fifty-eight years of age, and the perinæal operation had been unsuccessful.

In the following history, the dates and items of the earlier operations, I have taken from Cheselden, Heister, Frère Côme, Sharp, Baseilhac, Carpue, Belmas, Souberbeille, Humphrey, Günther, Dulles, Cooper, and Velpeau, with such information as I have been able to glean from other sources. The latter portion of the history, particularly that of the American operations, are given in Dr. Dulles's tables just as he has made them, not desiring in any way to interfere with his labors. No apology is needed for thus employing the work of others in matters of history, for it is astonishing to find in tracing the different writings of those interested in the subject how very minutely one author has followed another. In Belmas's book, which is the most comprehensive, I have found many items of interest, and this work, together with that of Côme, Günther, and Carpue, have been my chief guidance.

To those who desire to examine further the bibliography of suprapubic lithotomy, not only in regard to those who have operated, but also with reference to those who have written upon the subject, I would recommend a perusal of these works.

It is the opinion of some scholars and authors that the "high apparatus" can be carried back to Philagrius, who flourished shortly after Galen; he is reputed to have operated for a calculus impacted in the urethra, for he recommends the incision to be made "*superne juxta glandis magnitudinem.*" Samuel Cooper,† however, states that hypogastric lithotomy was first practiced

* Ranking's Abstract of the Medical Sciences, vol. xii, 1850, p. 130; art. 86.
† Surgical Dictionary, New York, Harper & Brother, 1854, p. 137.

in Paris in 1475 by Colot. The patient was a criminal, and was operated upon by permission of Louis XI. It is said that recovery took place in a fortnight. His claim to priority is denied by Velpeau,* who declares that Mr. Cooper had no grounds for the assertion, and that it is very uncertain what operation was performed by Colot.

There is also an idea prevalent among some antiquarian searchers, among whom is found one Nevermann, that the high operation for stone in the bladder might be traced to a period as remote as 1000 years B. C.; but in speaking on this very point Günther says that there can be no foundation for such an assertion, because the description of the operation in the *Ayur-Veda* is according " to the cut of Celsus." This, however, would scarcely be held as tenable, for Celsus himself may have copied from the Hindoos. Brockhaus, however, asserts that the *Ayur-Veda* is not older than B. C. 150. Others are of opinion that Atius, in the year 550, performed the first operation. By general consent, however, priority belongs to Pierre Franco, who in 1561, according to Belmas† and Velpeau,‡ and 1560, according to Heister,§ resorted to suprapubic lithotomy with success at Lausanne. The method he resorted to was the old one of " cutting on the gripe," as it was called, transferred from the perinæum to the hypogastrium. He says his patient was operated upon " on the mons veneris, a little to one side and over the stone, while he raised up the last with his two fingers, which were in the fundament, and keeping it moreover under his control by means of the hands of an assistant, which made compression on the lower belly."

I find also that some surgeons have stated that Franco's incision was made transversely " parallel to and a short distance above the superior border of the pubes."‖

Franco, however, can scarcely be called an upholder of the method, for Heister states specifically, that he was moved more by the entreaties of the parents to rescue their child from misery than from any foregone conclusion of the superior merits of the operation. The patient was a boy, aged two years, and the stone was the size of a hen's egg, which he had been unable to extract from the perinæum.¶ Velpeau again corrects the latter portion of the statement, and avers that Franco had not previously cut the patient in the perinæum. Carpue states that the operation was performed " en deux temps."

Twenty years after, Franco's operation being in 1581, Rousset (Rossetus) described it and published a work in its favor, though he was never able to

---

* Velpeau, Operative Surgery, vol. iii, p. 947.
† Traité de la Cystotomie Suspubienne. Paris, 1827, p. 2.   ‡ Operative Surgery, vol. ii, p. 947.
§ Institutiones Chirurgicæ. D. Laurentii Heisteri, tom. ii, p. 927.
‖ Bernard and Huett's Manual of Operative Surgery. Van Buren & Isaacs, New York, 1857, p. 434.
¶ Tamesti enim primus ejusdem auctor feliciter eandem in puero bimulo, Lausannæ, A.D 1560, instituerat, propterea quod calculum qui ovum gallinæ æquabat, in perinæo educere non poterat. D. Laurentii Heisteri Institutiones Chirurgicæ, vol. ii, p. 926.

perform it, on account of the death of Henry III, who, as Velpeau says, "had promised to assign him three or four criminals for experimentation."* This book was afterward translated into Latin under the name *De Partis Cæsaris*.

The method recommended by Rousset was to fill the bladder with water, milk, barley-water, or other fluid, to distend it sufficiently above the pubis; then to place a ligature around the penis, or to have that organ squeezed tightly by an assistant, to prevent the escape of the fluid. A razor was used to divide the integument and fascia, and a concave bistoury was then introduced just above the symphysis pubis; into this puncture a lenticular bistoury was inserted and the incision completed from below, upwards. The calculus was then to be extracted with the fingers if possible, if not, by means of a suitable scoop.

But to return. After Franco's operation a long time must have elapsed without much attention being given to hypogastric lithotomy, for the next record is not until the year 1635, when Mercier defended the operation in a thesis of N. Piètre. Of this Guy-Paten states that he (Piètre) performed the operation several times in 1635.†

Piètre died in 1649, and was the first to recommend lifting the bladder by means of a sound or catheter.‡

In the year 1681, we are informed by Tollet, that Bonnet (Bonnetus) practiced the high operation at the Hôtel Dieu, and that it was witnessed by the celebrated Petit. These records, however, were discredited by John Douglass, of whom more will be spoken; but Belmas§ and others are of the opinion that Douglass, desiring to be considered the reviver of the operation after Franco, was therefore disposed to ignore any claims advanced by others to priority in its performance.

In the year 1694 Proby, a surgeon of Dublin, resorted to the high operation, after the method of Franco, to remove a bodkin from the bladder of a girl.|| Dupuytren¶ is of opinion that this should scarcely be classed as a lithotomy, and perhaps it should more properly come under the head of hypogastric section. In 1710 John Groenvelt, a Dutch lithotomist, who afterwards, under the name of Greenfield, practiced surgery in London, informs us, in the second edition of his works, that he was obliged to resort to the high operation in a difficult case of stone in the bladder.

A few years after this, viz., in 1718, James Douglass, a Scotch anatomist, read a memorial on "The High Operation for Stone," before the Royal Society

---

* Loc. cit., vol. iii, p. 947.

† Belmas, p. 2. The title of this Thesis was "Questio medico-chirurgica quam præside Piètre tuebatur." Le Mercier. Paris, 1635.

‡ Günther. Operation am Becken, p. 308.

§ Belmas, loc. cit., p. 3; also Velpeau, vol. iii, p. 947.

|| Philosophical Transactions, vol. xxii, as quoted by Carpue.

¶ Lithotomie. Thèse, par G. Dupuytren. Paris, 1812, p. 35.

of London, in which, from inference drawn from the anatomical relations of the parts, he strongly advocated the method. It was but one year after the reading of this paper (1719) that John Douglass, his brother, performed his first operation at the Westminster Hospital, and followed it by a second in the same year, and three others in 1720. It is said that Douglass, believing himself to be the reviver of the operation, called it after his own name, and published in the same year a work upon the subject.* His method was somewhat similar to that advised by Rossetus, though he discarded the razor and substituted in its place the bistoury. He moderately injected the bladder, and made the incision in the viscus with the same instrument without a previous puncture.† He appears, in his anxiety to be considered foremost in resuscitating the method, to have discredited or ignored the labors of those who had given attention to the subject since Franco's time, and to have endeavored to introduce his method into the hospitals, as an operation of his own, bearing his own name. According to Belmas, however, he met with decided opposition on the part of the surgeons of his time, they refusing to perform the high operation in the public charities. The only exception to this was Cheselden, who being attracted by the feasibility of the procedure proclaimed his convictions in its favor, for which service Douglass dedicated to him a panegyric in Latin.

In the year 1721, Paul, of St. Thomas's Hospital, performed four successful suprapubic lithotomies. The first two of these are mentioned by Belmas and Günther,‡ but the whole four are said to have been successful by Holmes.§ Humphreys, on the other hand, informs us that two died.||

Cheselden having become the champion of this method, performed his first operation in 1722, and in 1723 published a dissertation on the subject.¶ In Cheselden's Appendix** to *The Anatomy of the Human Body*, will be found the following: "The next season, it being my term in St. Thomas's, I resumed the high way, *and cutting nine with success*, it came again into vogue. After that every lithotomist practiced it." The method he adopted was to first inject the bladder with some bland fluid, in quantity equal to that of urine, which the patient could retain in his bladder, and after having incised the integument in the mesial line, to cut the bladder from above downward. The success of Cheselden aroused the bitter animosity of Douglass, who accused him of appropriating to himself the honor that should belong rightly to the reviver of the operation. He wrote a diatribe against Cheselden, which contrasted

---

* Lithotomia Douglassiana, with a Course of Operations. London, 1720.
† Velpeau, loc. cit., p. 948, vol. iii.
‡ Loc. cit., p. 5.   § System of Surgery, vol. iv, p. 1075. Also Carpue, p. 160.
|| Trans. Pro. Med. and Surg. Ass., 1850, p. 103.
¶ A Treatise on the High Operation for Stone. With seventeen copper-plates. London, 1723.
** The Anatomy of the Human Body. By W. Cheselden. Ninth Edition, with forty copper-plates, London, 1773. Chapter VI. A Short Historical Account of Cutting for the Stone, p. 327.

singularly with his previous essay in praise of the great surgeon. It is well known that, shortly after, this distinguished surgeon abandoned the "high apparatus," and concentrated his labors upon the lateral perinæal method, with which to this day his name is inseparably connected. In giving his reasons for this he states that because "the peritoneum often being burst or cut, and the bladder itself was burst from injecting too much water, which generally proved fatal in a day or two, ... and that the urine lying continually in the wound retarded the cure," he had hoped to find a better method. It is remarkable, however, that a little further on he uses this peculiar language: "Though the operation came into universal discredit, I must declare it as my opinion, *that it is much better than the old way*, to which they all returned except myself, who would not have left the ' high way ' but for the hope I had of a better."*

In the year 1723 Heister made his first operation. It is so interesting that I may give the account of the case in his own words. He says: "Led by the same necessity as Franco and Greenfield, on April 17th, 1723, I did not hesitate to adopt this new and approved method of lithotomy, in the case of a man aged thirty years. I had ineffectually attempted to remove a part of the calculus by the ordinary method through an incision made in the perinæum, because it had fallen back into the pit, or diverticulum of the bladder, which has often been observed by others. On the following day, many students of medicine and surgery being present, without filling the bladder (which in cases of this kind cannot be done by reason of the lower wound) a cut was made over the pubes and in the body of the bladder, according to the directions of Rossetus and Douglass, by means of a curved scalpel. The wound was then extended above and below by means of a lentil-shaped instrument, and I withdrew the calculus easy enough with my fingers."†

In the same year, Prœbisch, a surgeon in the Prussian army, successfully performed epicystotomy on a child, twelve years of age, and reported a second recovery after an operation by Rungius, on a male patient, aged twenty-six years. ▪ According to Günther, this operation was performed in 1727, at Königsberg. In October of the same year, MacGill performed suprapubic lithotomy, and communicated his method with his case to Dr. Campbell, which is mentioned in Cheselden's book. In February, Thornhill, of Bristol, operated by this method, and soon followed it by others, so that he was enabled to publish sixteen cases, of which three died. There is a little discrepancy to be found in the dates of Thornhill's operations, between Belmas and Humphrey. The former‡ making the date as above given, while the latter, in his tables, gives three operations in the year 1722,§ in which Günther agrees. It is quite

---

* Loc. cit., chapter vi, Anatomy of the Human Body.
† Institutiones Chirurgicæ, vol. ii, p. 929. Belmas, loc. cit., p. 5.   ‡ Loc. cit., p. 6.
§ Transactions of the Provincial Medical and Surgical Association, 1850, vol. xvii, p. 103.

remarkable that this surgeon should have seen and treated such a number of cases in so short a period of time. Carpue tells us that Middleton, of whom we shall speak directly, was present at all of Thornhill's operations.

Pye, of Bristol, made his first epicystotomy in 1722, and followed it by three others, in 1724. Of the four, three died, one died of sloughing, one of cancer, and the third of kidney disease, probably pyo-nephrosis.

In 1724, James Roberts, who like many others of the present day, was rather unfavorably impressed with suprapubic lithotomy, was obliged to perform it, and the case terminating successfully, he then (and I trust his example may be followed by the surgeons of our time) altered his views and became a partisan of the " high apparatus."

In the year 1726, Sermes, a surgeon of Amsterdam, was as unfortunate as Pye, and wrote a work entirely condemning hypogastric lithotomy.

It is to him that priority is due in making the supplementary incision below the pubes, which is often attributed to Côme. It was for practicing this additional cut, or as it was called the "button-hole" incision, that he was persecuted by the profession, and even condemned by the tribunal of his country.*

In the year 1727, John Middleton published a short essay on the subject,† which contains also a letter from Dr. MacGill to Dr. Douglass. It is probable from this that Dr. MacGill, who is mentioned above, communicated with both Cheselden and Douglass his ideas and experience with the high apparatus. Middleton's book I have not been able to procure.

In the same year Colot, who was appointed by the French Parliament to investigate the high operation, made a report most adverse to it, in which he declared that its very contemplation inspired him with horror. He, however, states that Turbier, professor of surgery in Paris, saved, by epicystotomy, the life of a man, who was brought to the brink of the grave, by the presence of a calculus obstructing the neck of the bladder. In the year 1727, Sénac recorded two successful operations, and in the same year, 1728, Morand, or in 1727, according to Belmas—declared himself an advocate for the hypogastric section. His first operation was unsuccessful, the patient being a paralyzed old man, but as an offset to his fatal case he introduces a successful one of Berrier, and not being discouraged, still upheld the method.

It is interesting here to note a fact that Rameau, a surgeon of Montpellier, most severely criticised Morand for his adherence to hypogastric lithotomy, and that in his work may be found a careful description of the urethra, and the entrance thereto by *straight* instruments.‡

* Velpeau, loc. cit., vol. iii, p. 954.

† Lithotomy by a New Method above the Pubes, to which is added a letter from Dr. MacGill to Dr. Douglass.

‡ The title of Rameau's essay is, Réflexions en forme de lettre, ou Analyse de la dissertation de M. Morand, sur la taille au haut appareil. Amsterdam, 1729. *Vide* Belmas, p. 10.

Morand's operation differed but little from that of his predecessors, excepting that he directed the patient to lie with the hips elevated above the shoulders, the legs being secured to the bedposts. He also disapproved of elevating the bladder by means of injections, and recommends that the left forefinger be hooked and inserted into the upper angle of the wound, to prevent the bladder from slipping behind the pubic bones.

Morand's book was first published in 1728, and afterward in 1749, and Carpue mentions a fact which it is important to remember in regard to the statistics of the operation.* It is this, that Morand in speaking of Berrier's operating in 1727, remarked, "that he could give the history of forty operations, out of which thirty-five recovered."† It is well known that Humphrey, in his tables, which have been carefully examined, omits the operations of Frère Côme, and of a person he calls Maunde, and that Dulles states that in his classification, which formed the subject of his Thesis (but which has never been published), he also omits Maunde. Holmes also quotes from Humphrey to the same effect. To my mind, there has been an error in the reading of the manuscript, or of the proof, for "Morand" could easily be mistaken for "Maunde," and as the figures are exactly the same, it is probable that the error occurred in this manner. If Carpue makes "Bernier" read for Berrier, and Holmes makes Souberveille read for Souberbéille, and MacGill read Malgill, and Dupuytren makes Thornhill read Fornhill, why may not Maunde be meant for Morand?

In the year 1727, Senff made three suprapubics with two successes, and in 1728, Hildanus, in Switzerland, made the operation once, and in 1729, H. Hess resorted to it. It was in this year that Côme entered the order of the Bernardine Monks. Quite a period then elapsed without much attention being paid to the operation. Occasionally, however, surgeons were found taking an interest in "the high apparatus," among whom are Kulmus, in 1732, and Le Cat, in 1735. The latter proposed a method somewhat different from that of those who had preceded him, and following the suggestion of Thebaut that the abdominal and bladder wound should be incised at once, he invented an instrument to fulfil these indications. He named it a cystome bistoury. He performed the operation successfully, and communicated his ideas to the Royal College of Surgeons in London.

In 1755 Hempel operated with success, and in 1756 a surgeon of Copenhagen, named Heuerman, also reports favorably of the procedure, but the appearance of Frère Côme, with his modifications and successes, in 1758, gave a fresh impetus to "the high apparatus." In 1799, the monk,‡ whose name before

---

* In Carpue's book there must have been a typographical error, for he mentions the name Bernier, instead of Berrier, as referred to by Belmas, Dulles, Humphrey.

† History of the High Operation for Stone. By J. C. Carpue, F.R.S. London, 1819, p. 123.

‡ Carpue, p. 159.

he entered the monastery was Jean Baseilhac, had performed a hundred supra-pubic lithotomies with but nineteen deaths. Some declare that this remarkable man was entirely unlettered, a fact which is untrue. This ecclesiastic was born in the year 1703 in the parish of Poyestruc, near Tarbes. His record as a medical man was good, both his grandfather and father being surgeons. In 1722 he went to Lyons and placed himself under the instruction of Baseilhac, the elder, who enjoyed a high reputation. He entered college in 1729, and was elected professor in 1740. In 1799 he published his account of the high operation for stone in the bladder, which had fallen into disrepute since the time of Morand. To those desiring to read an interesting account of his life, as also of that of Frère Jacques, a work, by his nephew, is still extant in our libraries.* The hundred operations of hypogastric lithotomy of Frère Côme, with loss of only nineteen, to which allusion has just been made, are proverbial; but the fact is not generally known that in his own works, which have been carefully examined, he records but eighty-two of these cases; the balance being given by his nephew, Paschal Baseilhac, in the book to which reference has already been made.

In confirmation of this I insert here a short translation from the work in question. "Frère Côme, in his treatise on the High Operation on both sexes, gives a list of the cases in which he had operated by this method, down to the date of his publication, in 1779, from which it appears that his new method is more advantageous for females than for males; since out of his forty-six female cases, thirty-nine were cured, and only about one-sixth died. Whereas, he reports in the same work that he had operated on thirty-six male patients, and had lost eight of them—a mortality of almost one-quarter. Since the date at which this list was published he operated, down to his death in July, 1781, on five males and thirteen females, whose names and addresses, taken from his own register, are in my possession; making altogether forty-one males, and fifty-nine females, or a grand total of one hundred operated on, of whom there died ten males and nine females, or nineteen in all, while eighty-one were cured. Frère Côme would certainly not have lost so many if he could have profited by the experience, in regard to the new method, gained during the last period of his life, and if he had enjoyed better conveniences for treatment in his own infirmary, where three-fourths of his operations were performed. As he received no assistance from the government, this devoted man had to rely wholly on what his wealthy patients gave him, and on charitable contributions, which enabled him to provide proper food and attendance for scarcely thirty out of the multitude he admitted. Had he possessed the means, his wards would have been more roomy, and he would have employed trained nurses for

* Eloge Historique de Frère Côme, De La Taille Laterale et celle de l'hypogastric ou Haut Appareil. Par Paschal Baseilhac, p. 77.

3

night service, instead of girls, who could scarcely keep awake after the house-
hold labors of the day. We see that he was less successful in the case of males
than that of females, yet out of the total number of both sexes on which he
performed the high operation, rather more than four-fifths were cured, a far
better result than was yielded by the *grand appareil*, from which usually
about one-third recovered."

It may also be well to remark here that although very many writers on this
subject, especially his own countrymen, give the Fueillant ecclesiastic the name
Côme, yet others, among whom we find Dulles and Günther, spell the
name Cosme. Côme is supposed by many to have introduced the *sonde-à-dard*,
and the incision below the pubes, but, as has already been mentioned, Sermes
first proposed the idea of the button-hole incision, and the introduction of
sounding instruments into the perinæum to facilitate the performance of the
operation. The real inventor, however, of the "sonde," although many have
proposed and effected modifications of it, was M. Pallucci,* who in 1750
brought it to the notice of the profession. However, it is not the name of the
inventor, but that of the promulgator and utilizer, which generally descends to
posterity.

The name of Morton will always be associated with ether anæsthesia, and
that of Sayre with the suspension apparatus and plaster jacket; so will the
sond-à-darde be remembered as the instrument of Frère Côme. His method of
employing the "sonde" was rather peculiar. He first introduced a staff into
the bladder; an incision about an inch in length in the perinæum, similar to
that practiced in median lithotomy, was then made. A second cut was then
carried into the membranous urethra. A grooved director was passed into the
bladder through the last-named wound, and the staff immediately withdrawn.
The sonde was, by means of the groove in the director, slid into the bladder.
So soon as this was accomplished, the abdominal parietes were incised. A
trocar, in which there was a concealed bistoury, was next passed into the linea
alba close to the pubes, and the blade of the knife then started from its sheath
toward the handle of the instrument, while its other end remained stationary ;
thus the linea alba was incised from below upwards. If necessary, this incision
was enlarged by means of a probe-pointed bistoury, shielded in front by the
finger, to push the peritoneum out of the way in case the knife should slip.
The incision thus being made, and the bladder brought into view, the sonde
was pressed up against the anterior wall of the bladder, and held there with the
thumb and forefinger, while an assistant pushed up the stilette, and thus opened
the viscus; a curved, sharp-pointed bistoury was then introduced into the groove
in the stilette, and the bladder cut from above downward, oft-times nearly to

---

* Günther, Operationem am Becken, p. 308.

its neck. The fingers were immediately introduced into the wound, and the bladder held up by them, while the sonde-à-dard was withdrawn by an assistant. As an extra precaution against the bladder falling behind the pubes, a hook was introduced into its upper extremity, and the stone readily withdrawn with forceps. An elastic catheter was then passed into the wound through the opening previously made in the perinæum.*

The success of Côme was certainly remarkable, and is admitted by the generality of inquiries into the statistics of the operation. It is therefore quite unfair to omit these cases from the tables prepared by Mr. Humphreys,† simply because the results were so favorable. That certain operations are more successful in the hands of one surgeon than another, is a peculiar and rather unpleasant fact in surgery. What might be thought of the statistics of Mr. Keith in ovariotomy as compared with other skilful operators? It would be almost supposable that at a future day, as some one is looking up the history of ovariotomy, that the wonderful success of the great surgeon should be ignored because his results were so surprisingly successful.

In 1784, Pascal Baseilhac performed epicystotomy on a girl, aged eighteen years. His work, as already mentioned, records the additional fifteen cases of his uncle and preceptor, and also analyzes and criticises other cases and the operation in general. In 1773, Le Blanc performed the operation, recommending it for large calculi. In the year 1786 Lassus, as recorded by Cooper‡ and Belmas,§ attempted lithotomy in the perinæum with Hawkins's gorget, but being unable to remove the calculus, he had recourse to the suprapubic method with success. About the same period Deguise was obliged to resort to the "high apparatus" to remove a stone which he had fruitlessly attempted to extract through the perinæum. In this year also, according to Günther, Espiaux also had recourse to the operation. In 1790 the method was resorted to by Lauvejat to remove a stone which materially obstructed labor. Mursima, in 1797, or about that time, employed the hypogastric method on account of an obstinate stricture.

In the year 1802 another renowned operator appears upon the field as a champion, at all events for a time, of the hypogastric method of removing calculi from the bladder, viz., Dupuytren. Belmas states specifically that he had frequently seen this distinguished operator remove large stones by this method. His thesis, presented with his application for the chair of Surgery,

---

* Nouvelle Méthode d'extraire la pierre de la vessie urinaire par dessus la pubes, qu'on nomme vulgairement le Haut Appareil, dans l'un et l'autre sexe, sans le secours d'aucun fluide retenu ne forcé, dans la vessie. Par F. Côme. Paris, 1779.

† Humphreys, Transactions Provincial Medical and Surgical Association, vol. v. p. 104, 1861. Quoted by Holmes, vol. iv, p. 1076, and Dulles's American Jour. of the Medical Sciences.

‡ Surgical Dictionary, p. 137.   § Loc. cit., page 12.

in the Hôtel Dieu, was upon lithotomy, and its varied methods.* He also in this work alludes to the fact, that the perinæal incision might often be followed by disastrous consequences.

In 1808 Scarpa records a successful case, and made a modification of the sonde-à-dard, which consisted in having the groove in the stilette of sufficient depth to allow the introduction of the bistoury above it, and being so arranged that the end of the instrument always must remain in the bladder, while the point of the stilette is thrust through the vesical wall.

It is worthy of remark also in this place, that this distinguished surgeon regarded the additional wound in the perinæum as unnecessary, and that in 1812 Dupuytren also followed his example, declaring that "the sonde, or other instrument to raise and perforate the bladder, could be introduced by way of the urethra." Between the years 1809 and 1816, Vacca Belinghieri performed the operation six times.

In the year 1818, Kirby, in order to remove a probe or sound which had accidentally slipped into the bladder, opened that viscus above the pubes, and in 1820 Krouse made use of the high apparatus. In the year 1819, Carpue wrote his book, which contains a very clear description of the steps of the operation as it was done at that time. He first saw Souberbielle perform it, in 1817, on M. De Walville, at the Hôtel des Invalides. He writes as follows :†

"First, an incision is made through the integument of the perinæum, and a small incision into the membranous part of the urethra; a director is introduced into the bladder, upon the staff; the staff is withdrawn; the sonde-à-dard is introduced upon the director into the bladder; the director is now withdrawn; the sonde-à-dard is held by an assistant. An incision is made, three or four inches in length, through the integuments of the abdomen. The trocar-bistoury is passed through the linea alba, close to the posterior part of the pubis. The concealed blade is opened, by means of which the lower part of the linea alba is divided. A probe-pointed bistoury is introduced, through the opening which has been made by the concealed bistoury, into the lower part of the linea alba, and the incision is continued by means of this instrument. The operator takes the sonde-à-dard from the assistant with his right hand, and pushes it forward, by which means he elevates the bladder above the pubis. The assistant now holds the sonde-à-dard, and the surgeon with his right hand pushes the stilette (which is contained in the canula of the sonde-à-dard) through the anterior part of the bladder; he takes hold of the end of the stilette with his left hand, and passes a probe-pointed bistoury along the groove (which is in the anterior part of the stilette), and makes an incision in the su-

---

* Lithotomie, Thèse, soutenue publiquement dans l'Amphithéatre de la Faculté de Médecine de Paris; en Présence des Juges du concours, le 29 Janvier, 1812, par G. Dupuytren, Docteur en Chirurgie, Chirurgien en chef adjoint à l'Hôtel-Dieu de Paris, chef des travaux anatomiques de la Faculté, à Paris, MDCCCXII.

† History of the High Operation for Stone, by J. C. Carpue, F.R.S., M.R.C.S., London, 1819.

perior anterior part of the bladder. He passes the index finger of his left hand into the bladder, by means of which he supports it. The stilette is withdrawn from the canula of the sonde-à-dard, which is now lowered and held by an assistant; the operator introduces the suspensor of the bladder, which is held by an assistant. The stone is now to be withdrawn with the finger and thumb, which if small is done with great ease. If the bladder is large, a finger is introduced per rectum, by which the bladder is elevated, and the stone more readily found. If the stone should be in an excavation, and the bladder is not of very large size, it may be discovered with the finger, by means of which the surgeon will know whether a scoop or what kind of forceps is indicated. If the stone should be very large, Frère Côme's forceps must be used. If the stone should adhere to the bladder, or be contained in a cyst, the means used by M. Baseilhac and Sir Everard Home should be resorted to. When the stone has been extracted, Dr. Souberbeille introduces a silver wire through the canula of the sonde-à-dard, and passes it through the wound made in the linea alba; this is held while the sonde-à-dard is withdrawn; a flexible gum catheter is now passed into the bladder, through the wound in the membranous part of the urethra, by means of this wire. The wire is now withdrawn. The catheter is confined in this situation, by means of tapes passed around the thighs and pelvis of the patient; a bladder is tied to it to receive the urine."

It is worthy of remark, in this place, that after the year 1825 Souberbeille performed the operation without the perinæal incision,* but Dulles states that the supposition is that most of his operations were made with the perinæal cut; but as the majority of the recorded cases were after 1822–1825, this must be an error. In 1835 Souberbeille made his report to the Académie Royal 'de Médecine of fifty cases of the operation with but four deaths;† but these cases it must be remembered were not all suprapubic lithotomies. From a careful examination of his record it is found that of these there were thirty-nine "suspubienne" and eleven lateral. It may be as well also to remark here that Souberbeille begins his table with the year 1828, whereas he must have operated many times before, as I have discovered by the examination of Belmas's book, who even records cases operated upon as far back as 1796.

But to retrace the history for a moment. Sir Everard Home, at St. George's Hospital, performed the operation first on the 26th of May, 1820, and followed it with two others. He called his method a new one. He made an incision in the linea alba, and detached portions of the pyramidales at their insertion; the finger was then introduced behind the pubes and the bladder felt for. A silver catheter with an open end was passed into the bladder, and when the end was detected by the finger in the wound, a stilette was thrust

---

* Velpeau, Operative Surgery, vol. iii, p. 955.
† Mémoires de l'Académie Royal de Médecine, Paris, 1840.

upward through the bladder. The opening was then enlarged, the fundus of the bladder held up with the left hand, while the stone was extracted with the right hand.*.

In the year 1822 Deguise performed the operation once, and about the same time Dzondi resorted to it four times. Textor in 1823 essayed the operation after lateral lithotomy. In 1824 the first American suprapubic was made by Professor Gibson, of the University of Pennsylvania. In his Surgery† he states that he followed the method of Sir E. Home, and removed two calculi. The patient went on so well that Gibson says: "He insisted upon the catheter being withdrawn, contrary to very strict injunctions which I left with him, and in consequence soon after perished from peritoneal inflammation induced by a fusion of urine in the cavity of the pelvis."

Between the years 1825 and 1830, the following surgeons had recourse to the method, viz.: Hutchinson, Ballingall, Amussat (7) ; Krimer, with his remarkable case of tremendous calculus ; Baudens, three operations ;‡ Roux, in 1827 ;§ Crozat, of Tours, who in performing the operation cut into the peritonæum, but the patient (a woman) made a good recovery ;‖ George Bell, on a man aged eighty,¶ who recovered. About the same time that Roux was operating in Paris, Carpenter and McClellan performed their operations in America. For the balance of the American epicystotomies, with their dates and references, I refer the reader to Dr. Dulles's tables, which are given entire, knowing how much time and patience must have been expended upon them. The first table extends from Gibson's case in 1824 to Gidding's in 1844,** and his second comprises the operations of ten years, between 1867 and 1877.†† In Dr. Dulles's tables, however, I find he has overlooked an epicystotomy performed by Hammer, of St. Louis.‡‡ Gunther gives the following cases :

Delpech, in 1831, two operations ; Leroy d'Etiolles, 1834, one operation ; Segur, 1835, three operations ; Moulini, 1839, one operation ; Souberbeille, to which allusion has already been made ; Larrey, 1841, one operation ; Smith, 1841, one operation ; Nélaton, 1841, one operation ; Civiale five, 1841 to 1844 ; Segalas, 1844, one ; Gaillard, 1844, one ; Günther, from 1845, eight with success ; Paine, about 1848, one ; Olivarez, 1848, three ; Bruns, from 1848, three ; Langenbeck, from 1849, five ; Unger, 1850, one ; Schlobig, 1850, one ; Geinetz, 1850, one ; Staude, in 1854, four ; Schmid, 1856, two ; Stölle and Bezin, 1856, one ;

---

* Cooper's Surgical Dictionary, Article Lithotomy.
† Institutes and Practice of Surgery, by William Gibson, M.D., vol. ii, p. 231. Philadelphia, 1835.
‡ Günther, p. 306. Sabbatier, p. 249.   § Velpeau, vol. iii, p. 951.
‖ Velpeau, vol. iii, p. 951.   ¶ London Lancet, vol. ii, 1858, p. 663.
** American Journal of the Medical Sciences, 1875, p. 59.
†† American Journal of the Medical Sciences, 1878, p. 400.
‡‡ St. Louis Medical and Surgical Journal, 1865, p. 51.

Morlanne, 1856, one; Solzbeck, 1858, one. It is at this date that Günther's record closes.

M. Chauvel states that D'Almiera has since 1860 performed twenty-three operations.*

In 1861, Ash Wednesday, Sampson Gamgee, at the Queen's Hospital, in London, removed a good-sized calculus from a girl, aged eight years and nine months. The calculus weighed 305 grains, and measured 1⅝ inches in length, and 1¼ inches in breadth.†

Quite a remarkable case is recorded in 1862, by Dr. Chisholm, in which a man was shot in the crest of the ilium, and the bullet was removed by the suprapubic incision. In the same year Dr. McGue had a somewhat similar but unsuccessful case.‡

The following tables, showing the dates, the names of the operators, the size of the stone, etc., are offered to the profession, with the hope that they may assist in forming some idea of the history of this operation. The tables have been prepared with great care, and have taken considerable time. *They are, however, very far from being perfect, for several reasons; in the first place, there is often a discrepancy of a year to five years between the dates assigned by different authors for the performance of the operation.* Then again, the reports are very imperfect indeed, that is, in regard to the particulars of the operation, the size of the stone, and the result. Therefore, the only just method for arriving at the average mortality is to classify only those cases in which the results are given.

---

* Dictionnaire Encyclop. des Sciences Medicales, 1880, vol. **xxv**, p. 105.
† London Lancet, vol. ii, 1873, p. 807.
‡ Medical and Surgical History of the War of the Rebellion, vol. ii, p. 282.

CHAPTER II.*

TABLES OF SUPRAPUBIC LITHOTOMY.

It is necessary that these tables should be prefaced by a few remarks regarding the labors, in the same direction, of others whose work has necessarily come under observation ; and although in the previous chapter, most of the items of historical interest have been mentioned, yet there are a few others, bearing especially upon the statistics of the operation, which ought to be noticed in this place.

One of the most important of these is the fact that M. Chauvel, in the twenty-fifth volume of the *Dictionnaire Encyclopedique des Sciences Médicales* for 1880, falls into a curious error in reporting seven hundred and eighty-five operations of suprapubic lithotomy. He adds the cases collected by Belmas, Carpue, Günther, Humphreys, Souberbeille, Gross, etc., as if the numbers mentioned by each of these surgeons represented separate and distinct cases, whereas it is very obvious that Humphreys's one hundred and four includes many of those of Belmas, Carpue, Gross, and those of Souberbeille, as well as those of other surgeons, and Dulles's three hundred and sixty-four, those previously mentioned, etc.

In the sixth edition of Mr. Coulson's *Diseases of the Bladder*, several pages are devoted to the subject, and the statistics of Dulles given as a basis of comparison with the other methods. The data of suprapubic lithotomy, however, are for the most part scattered generally throughout the field of surgical literature. This will account in a great degree for the many blanks that appear in the table in reference to the particulars of age, sex, and the cause of death. Nothing doubtful or unknown has been assumed, and only such accepted as authentic for which there was undoubted and trustworthy references.

No attempt to compile a full historical table of suprapubic lithotomy has ever before been offered to the profession, and in making the fresh effort in that direction we by no means claim to have succeeded in collecting all the cases upon whom this method has been employed, for there are several surgeons who are known to have recourse to this procedure, of whose cases no record has been obtained.

---

* This chapter has been prepared with great care, by E. Guernsey Rankin, A.M., M.D., to whom the author desires to return thanks for the labor necessarily involved in the preparation of such statistics, and also to Drs. Lilienthal, Freeman, Swift, and Wilcox, for their assistance in this direction.

	NAME.	DATE.	AGE.	SEX.	SIZE.	RESULT.	OBSERVATIONS.	REFERENCES.
1	Franco.	1560	2	M.	Hen's egg.	Recovered.	After failure of lateral lithotomy.	Velpeau, vol. iii, p. 947. Heister, vol. ii, p. 927. Franco, p. 139, et seq. Côme, p. 95. Günther, p. 305.
2	Petrie.	1635	..	..	. . .	Recovered.	. . . .	Belmas, p. 2. Coulson, p. 156.
3	Jean de Dot.	1651	..	M.	Goose egg.	Recovered.	Operated on himself.	Hyrtl, p. 293. Holden, p. 31.
4	Bonnet.	1681	..	..	. . .	Recovered.	. . . .	Belmas, p. 3. Velpeau, vol. iii, p. 947.
5	Proby.	1694	20	F.	. . .	Recovered.	Removed a bodkin.	Carpue, p. 68, et seq. Baseilhac, p. 315. Philos. Trans., vol. xxi, p. 1700. Humphrey, p. 103. Belmas, p. 3. Sabattier, vol. iv, p. 234. Günther, p. 33. Côme, p. 9. Coulson, p. 157. Velpeau, vol. iii, p. 947. Dict. Encyclop. des Sciences Med., 1881, vol. xxv, p. 95.
6	Greenfield.	1710	..	..	. . .	Recovered.	. . . .	Carpue, p. 68. Belmas, p. 4. Sabattier, vol. xii, p. 234. Humphrey, p. 103.
7	John Douglass	1719	17	M.	Small hen's egg.	Recovered.	. . . .	Carpue, p. 77, et seq. Holmes, vol. iv, p. 1075. Coulson, p. 157.
8	John Douglass.	1720	8	M.	Horse-chestnut.	Recovered.	. . . .	Baseilhac, p. 321. Günther, p. 306. Belmas, p. 4.
9	John Douglass.	1720	3	M.	Horse-chestnut.	Died.	Convulsions 15 hours after.	Philos. Trans., yrs. 1720–'22, vol. iii, p. 228, et seq. Humphrey, p. 103. Cheselden, p. 327.
10	John Douglass.	1720	4	..	Horse-chestnut.	Recovered.	Peritoneum wounded. Intestines protruded and replaced.	Günther (to the 9th case only), p. 340.
11	Paul.	1721	..	..	. . .	Recovered.	. . . .	Carpue, p. 160. Holmes, vol. iv, p. 1075.
12	Paul.	1721	..	..	. . .	Recovered.	. . . .	Belmas, pp. 4 and 5. Günther, p. 306.
13	Paul.	1721 (about.)	..	..	. . .	Recovered	. . . .	
14	Paul.	1721 (about.)	..	..	. . .	Recovered.	. . . .	NOTE.—The last two authors refer only to the first two cases of Mr. Paul.
15	Cheselden.	1722	7	M.	. . .	Recovered.	. . . .	Carpue, pp. 79 and 89. Belmas, p. 5. Humphrey, p. 105. Baseilhac, p. 32.
16	Cheselden.	1722	14	M.	. . .	Recovered.	. . . .	

4

	NAME.	DATE.	AGE.	SEX.	SIZE.	RESULT.	OBSERVATIONS.	REFERENCES.
17	Cheselden.	1722	14	M.	. . .	Recovered	. . . .	Cheselden, p. 327. Holmes, vol. iv, p. 1075. Günther, pp. 306 and 319.
18	Cheselden.	1722	12	M.	. . .	Recovered.	. . . .	"
19	Cheselden.	1722	9	M.	. . .	Recovered.	. . . .	"
20	Cheselden.	1722	18	M.	. . .	Died.	Suppuration; stone in kidney, and diarrhœa; death 25th day.	"
21	Cheselden.	1722	19	M.	. . .	Recovered.	. . . .	"
22	Cheselden.	1722	11	M.	. . .	Recovered.	. . . .	"
23	Cheselden.	1722	4	M.	. . .	Recovered.	. . . .	"
24	Thornhill.	1722	8	M.	. . .	Recovered.	. . . .	Carpue. pp. 93 and 104. Humphrey, p. 103. Belmas, p. 7. Holmes, vol. iv, p. 1075. Günther, pp. 306 and 341, refers to 13 cases only.
25	Thornhill.	1722	6	M.	. . .	Recovered.	. . . .	"
26	Thornhill.	1722	15	M.	. . .	Recovered.	. . . .	"
27	Thornhill.	1723	45	M.	. . .	Recovered.	. . . .	"
28	Thornhill.	1723	4	M.	Peach stone.	Recovered.	. . . .	"
29	Thornhill.	1723	48	M.	. . .	Recovered.	. . . .	"
30	Thornhill.	1723	14	M.	. . .	Died.	Gangrene of peritoneum; bladder found to be scirrhous; peritoneum wounded.	NOTE.—Belmas gives the date for Thornhill's first case as 1723.
31	Thornhill.	1723	13	M.	. . .	Died.	. . . .	"
32	Thornhill.	1723	18	M.	. . .	Recovered.	. . . .	"
33	Thornhill.	1724	5	M.	. . .	Recovered.	. . . .	"
34	Thornhill.	1724	55	M.	. . .	Recovered.	. . . .	"
35	Thornhill.	1724	..	..	. . .	Recovered.		"
36	Thornhill.	1724	..	..	. . .	Recovered.		"
37	Thornhill.	1724	..	..	. . .	Recovered.	. . . .	"
38	Thornhill.	1724	..	..	. . .	Died.	3d day of scirrhus of bladder.	"
39	Thornhill.	1724	..	..	. . .	Recovered.	. . . .	"
40	Pye.	1722	7	M.	Large.	Died.	Abscess and sloughing of wound; death on 11th day.	Carpue, pp. 87 to 193 and 159. Belmas, p. 7. Humphrey, p. 103. Holmes, vol. iv, p. 1075.
41	Pye.	1724	5	M.	Nutmeg.	Recovered.	. . . .	Günther, p. 306.
42	Pye.	1724	19	M.	Large.	Died.	Ulceration and scirrhus of bladder.	"

	NAME.	DATE.	AGE.	SEX.	SIZE.	RESULT.	OBSERVATIONS.	REFERENCES.
43	Pye.	1724	9	M.	Large.	Died.	Suppuration of kidney; 21st day.	Günther, p. 306.
44	Proebisch.	1723	12	M.	. . .	Recovered.	. . . .	Belmas, p. 6. Günther, pp. 306 and 341. According to the latter, this operation was performed 5 years later. Heister, vol. ii, p. 952.
45	Heister.	1723	30	M.	Large.	Died.	After failure with the lateral; abscess and dilatation of pelvis of kidney.	Carpue, pp. 110 and 115. Belmas, p. 5. Baseilhac, p. 325. Humphrey, p 103. Günther, p. 33.* Heister, vol. ii, pp. 929 and 30.
46	Heister.	1723	about) Adult	M.	. . .	Died.	7th day after, gangrene, suppurative peritonitis; abscess of omentum.	"
47	Heister.	1723	(about) 20	M.	. . .	Recovered.	. . . .	"
48	Macgill.	1723	Bet. 60 and 70	M.	2 stones, each ℥iv. ss.	Recovered.	. . . .	Carpue, pp. 10–110. Belmas, p. 6. Günther, pp. 309 and 340. Humphrey, p. 105. Holmes, vol. iv, p. 1075. Günther, p. 335. Günther, p. 306.
49	Macgill.	1723	13	M.	℥ij. ℥i.	Recovered.	Bladder was ruptured by injection. Cured. however, in 8 weeks.	"
50	Macgill.	1723	35	M.	℥v.	Died.	Stone not removed, being encysted.	"
51	Macgill.	1723	8	M.	Nutmeg.	Recovered.	. . . .	"
52	Rungius.	1723	26	. .	. . .	Recovered.	. . . .	Belmas, p. 6. Günther, p. 306.
53	Roberts.	1724	. .	. .	. . .	Recovered.	. . . .	Belmas, p. 7.
54	Sermes.	1726	. .	. .	. . .	Died.	. . . .	Günther, p. 319.
55	Sermes.	1726	. .	. .	. . .	Died.	. . . .	"
56	Sermes.	1726	. .	. .	. . .	Died.	. . . .	"
57	Sermes.	. . .	. .	. .	. . .	Recovered.	. . . .	"
58	Sermes.	. . .	. .	. .	. . .	Recovered.	. . . .	"
59	Sermes.	1726	. .	. .	. . .	Recovered.	. . . .	"
60	Sermes.	. . .	. .	. .	. . .	Recovered.	. . . .	"
61	Sermes.	. . .	. .	. .	. . .	Recovered.	. . . .	"
62	Sermes.	. . .	. .	. .	. . .	Recovered.	. . . .	"
63	Sermes.	. . .	. .	. .	. . .	Recovered.	. . . .	"

* Günther, p. 17, Der Hohe Steinschn tt. L ipsic, 1851.

	NAME.	DATE.	AGE.	SEX.	SIZE.	RESULT.	OBSERVATIONS.	REFERENCES.
64	Sermes.	. . .	. .	. .	. . .	Recovered.	. . . .	Günther, p. 319.
65	Sermes.	. . .	. .	. .	. . .	Recovered.	. . . .	"
66	Sermes.	. . .	. .	. .	. . .	Recovered.	. . . .	"
67	Sermes.	. . .	. .	. .	. . .	Recovered.	. . . .	"
68	Sermes.	. . .	. .	. .	. . .	Recovered.	. . . .	"
69	Sermes.	. . .	. .	. .	. . .	Recovered.	. . . .	"
70	Morand.	1727 or '28 Belmas.	68	M.	$\mathfrak{Z}$v.	Died.	Paralytic; death on 43d day; urethritis and cystitis.	Velpeau, vol. iii, p, 947. Belmas, p. 10. Carpue, p. 115. Günther, p. 30.
71	Morand.	1727	4	M.	. . .	Recovered.	. . . .	Günther, p. 20, in Der Hohe-Steinschnitt. Leipsic, 1861.
72	Berrier.	1727	4	M.	Nutmeg.	Recovered.	. . . .	Belmas, p. 10. Humphrey, p. 105. Carpue, pp. 121 and 123. Günther, pp. 306 and 335. Velpeau, vol. iii, p. 947.
73	Turbier.	1727	Adult	M.	. . .	Recovered.	. . . .	Belmas, p. 9.
74	Senac.	1727	. .	. .	. . .	Recovered.	. . . .	Belmas, p. 9.
75	Senac.	1727	. .	. .	. . .	Recovered.	. . . .	"
76	Senff.	1727	. .	. .	. . .	Died.	. . . .	Günther, in Der Hohe Steinschnitt, p. 19.
77	Senff.	1727	. .	. .	. . .	Recovered.	. . . .	"
78	Senff.	1727	. .	. .	. . .	Recovered.	. . . .	"
79	Hildanus.	1728	. .	F.	. . .	Recovered.	. . . .	Günther, in Der Hohe Steinschnitt, p. 21.
80	Hempil.	1755	. .	. .	. . .	Recovered.	. . . .	Günther, in Der Hohe Steinschnitt, p. 22.
81	Hempil.	1755	. .	. .	. . .	Recovered.	. . . .	"
82	Heuermann.	1755	12	M.	. . .	Recovered.	. . . .	Günther, p. 306.
83	Unknown.	1758	Adult	F.	. . .	Died.	3d day, nucleus was a pin.	Poulet, vol. ii, p. 235.
84	Côme.	1758	60	F.	. . .	Died.	Abscess of kidney; death 44 hours after.	Côme, p. 82. The following 82 cases of Frère Côme are taken from his work, Nouvelle Methode pour la extraire la pierre. Paris, 1779; from pp. 79 to 173, as given for each case.
85	Côme.	1758	23	F.	$\mathfrak{Z}$iii., gr. i.	Died.	. . . .	Côme, p. 84.
86	Côme.	1759	27	F.	. . .	Recovered.	. . . .	" p. 85.

	NAME.	DATE.	AGE.	SEX.	SIZE.	RESULT.	OBSERVATIONS.	REFERENCES.
87	Côme.	1759	7	F.	Hen's egg.	Recovered.	. . . .	Frère Côme, p. 85.
88	Côme.	1760	64	F.	. . .	Recovered.	. . . .	" p. 87.
89	Côme.	1760	25	F.	Walnut.	Recovered.	. . . .	" p. 89.
90	Côme.	1761	17	F.	Walnut.	Recovered.	. . . .	" p. 90.
91	Côme.	1761	5	F.	Large pigeon's egg.	Recovered.	. . . .	" p. 90.
92	Côme.	1761	6 or 7	F.	. . .	Recovered.	. . . .	" p. 91.
93	Côme.	1761	26	F.	Hen's egg.	Recovered.	. . . .	" pp. 91-92.
94	Côme.	1762	3½	F.	Chestnut.	Recovered.	. . . .	" p. 94.
95	Côme.	1762	27	F.	. . .	Died.	17 days after, of pleurisy; abscess in vagina.	
96	Côme.	1762	4½	F.	Walnut.	Recovered.	. . . .	" p. 96.
97	Côme.	1763	55	F.	Stone broken in fragments.	Recovered.	. . . .	" p. 99.
98	Côme.	1764	60	F.	. . .	Recovered.	Size not mentioned; stone soft.	" pp. 99-100.
99	Côme.	1764	60	F.	. . .	Recovered.	. . . .	" pp. 100-101.
100	Côme.	1764	49	F.	Not given.	Died.	7th day, extravasation of blood into surrounding tissue, and internal hemorrhage; left kidney much softened.	" pp. 102-103.
101	Côme.	1766	43	F.	3 stones.	Recovered.	2 flat and long; one, size of a hen's egg.	" pp. 103-105.
102	Côme.	1766	9	F.	Hen's egg.	Recovered.	. . . .	" pp. 103-105.
103	Côme.	1767	56	F.	ʒiv, gr. ii.	Recovered.	. . . .	" p. 106.
104	Côme.	1767	28	F.	Medium.	Recovered.	. . . .	" p. 106.
105	Côme.	1767	45	F.	Hen's egg shape.	Died.	. . . .	" p. 105.
106	Côme.	1767	59	F.	. . .	Recovered.	. . . .	" p. 107.
107	Côme.	1768	4 & 8 mos.	F.	. . .	Recovered.	. . . .	" p. 108.
108	Côme.	1768	62	F.	Rupture of bladder.	Recovered.	. . . .	" p. 108.
109	Côme.	1768	9	F.	Walnut.	Died.	9th day after infiltration of blood into the abdomen. Bladder walls a finger thick; hemorrhagic exudation in left pleura; thickened intestinal wall.	" p. 112.
110	Côme.	1769	8	F.	Hen's egg.	Recovered.	. . . .	" p. 115.

	NAME.	DATE.	AGE.	SEX.	SIZE.	RESULT.	OBSERVATIONS.	REFERENCES.
111	Côme.	1769	35	F.	. . .	Recovered.	. . . .	Frère Côme, p. 113.
112	Côme.	1769	12	F.	. . .	Recovered.	. . . .	" p. 116.
113	Côme.	1769	5	F.	. . .	Died.	Helminthiasis 12 days after.	" p. 118.
114	Côme.	1769	36	F.	. . .	Died.	Pyonephrosis.	" p. 119.
115	Côme.	1770	. .	F.	. . .	Died.	Stone encysted; cystitis, ulceration of bladder, pelvic cellulitis.	" p. 120.
116	Côme.	1772	72	F.	Hen's egg.	Recovered.	. . . .	" p. 123.
117	Côme.	1772	Adult	F.	Hen's egg.	Recovered.	Patient had suffered three years; age not given.	" p. 124.
118	Côme.	1773	39	F.	. . .	Recovered.	. . . .	" p. 124.
119	Côme.	1773	40	F.	. . .	Recovered.	. . . .	" p. 125.
120	Côme.	1773	36	F.	. . .	Recovered.	. . . .	" p. 125.
121	Côme.	1773	27	F.	. . .	Recovered.	. . . .	" p. 125.
122	Côme.	1773	3	F.	. . .	Recovered.	. . . .	" p. 126.
123	Côme.	1774	9½	F.	. . .	Recovered.	. . . .	" p. 126.
124	Côme.	1774	40	F.	. . .	Recovered.	. . . .	" p. 126.
125	Côme.	1775	22	F.	. . .	Recovered.	. . . .	" p. 126.
126	Côme.	1776	9	F.	. . .	Recovered.	. . . .	" p. 127.
127	Côme.	1777	20	F.	. . .	Recovered.	. . . .	" p. 127.
128	Côme.	1777	34	F.	. . .	Recovered.	. . . .	" p. 127.
129	Côme.	1777	33	F.	. . . .	Recovered.	. . . .	" p. 127.
130	Côme.	1769	56	M.	Hen's egg; 2 stones.	Recovered.	. . . .	" p. 130.
131	Côme.	1769	16	M.	. . .	Cure.	. . . .	" p. 133.
132	Côme.	1769	70	M.	. . .	Died.	Peritonitis; hemorrhagic exudation into thoracic cavity.	" p. 135.
133	Côme.	1769	Adult	M.	. . .	Recovered.	. . . .	" p. 140.
134	Côme.	1769	9	M.	. . .	Recovered.	. . . .	" p. 142.
135	Côme.	1769	10	M.	. . .	Died.	5 days after peritonitis	" p. 142.
136	Côme.	1769	74	M.	℥iv.	Recovered.	. . . .	" p. 141.
137	Côme.	1771	24	M.	Hen's egg.	Recovered.	. . . .	" p. 144.
138	Côme.	1771	8	M.	. . .	Recovered.	. . . .	" p. 144.
139	Côme.	1771	15	M.	. . .	Recovered.	. . . .	" p. 152.

	NAME.	DATE.	AGE.	SEX.	SIZE.	RESULT.	OBSERVATIONS.	REFERENCES.
140	Côme.	1771	13	M.	Pigeon's egg.	Died.	Stone in the ureter; inflammation of kidney.	Frère Côme, p. 152.
141	Côme.	1771	Adult	M.	. . .	Died.	5th day after pelvic cellulitis; pleuritic exudation; pyemia.	" p. 155.
142	Côme.	1771	47	M.	℥vi., gr. ss.	Recovered.	. . . .	" p. 157.
143	Côme.	1773	70	M.	℥vii., gr.	Died.	Abscess of right kidney 23d day.	" p. 160.
144	Côme.	1773	33	M.	Hen's egg.	Recovered.	. . . .	" p. 161.
145	Côme.	1773	17	M	Broken pieces size of hen's egg.	Recovered.		
146	Côme.	1775	74	M.	. . .	Recovered.	. . . .	" p. 162.
147	Côme.	1775	76	M.	Hen's egg.	Recovered.	. . . .	" p. 163.
148	Côme.	1776	76	M.	2 stones size of hen's egg.	Recovered.	. . . .	" p. 163.
149	Côme.	1776	20	M.	Chestnut.	Recovered.	. . . .	" p. 164.
150	Côme.	1776	6	M.	. . .	Recovered.	. . . .	" p. 164.
151	Côme.	1776	25	M.	Large hen's egg.	Died.	Hemorrhage.	" p. 164.
152	Côme.	1776	7	M.	Hen's egg.	Recovered.	. . . .	" p. 165.
153	Côme.	1776	22	M.	. . .	Recovered.	. . . .	" p. 165.
154	Côme.	1776	17	M.	. . . .	. . . .	Stone was fixed and extracted with forceps.	" p. 165.
155	Côme.	1777	12	M.	. . .	Recovered.	. . . .	" p. 167.
156	Côme.	1777	61	M.	. . .	Recovered.	. . . .	" p. 168.
157	Côme.	1777	66	M.	. . .	Recovered.	. . . .	" p. 168.
158	Côme.	1777	45	M.	. . .	. . . .		" p. 169.
159	Côme.	1778	. .	M.	Hen's egg.	Recovered.	. . . .	" p. 169.
160	Côme.	1778	30	M.	. . .	Recovered.	. . . .	" p. 170.
161	Côme.	1778	18	M.	. . .	Recovered.	. . . .	" p. 170.
162	Côme.	1778	69	M.	. . .	Died, 9 days.	Pelvis of kidney full of pus and hydatids.	" p. 170.
163	Côme.	1778	11	M.	Walnut.	Died.	Pyemia.	" p. 172.
164	Côme.	1778	10	M.	Pigeon's egg.	Recovered.	. . . .	" p. 172.
165	Côme.	1778	42	M.	Turkey egg.	Recovered.	. . . .	" p. 173.
166	Côme.	1780	. .	F.	. . .	Recovered.	. . . .	Baseilhac, p. 62.

	NAME.	DATE.	AGE.	SEX.	SIZE.	RESULT.	OBSERVATIONS.	REFERENCES.
167	Côme.			F.	. . .	Recovered.	. . . .	From No. 167 to 183 are the cases mentioned by Pascal Baseilhac. There is no direct reference to the cases, merely a general summary of the sexes of the patients and the number of recoveries, from which these data are computed.
168	Côme.			F.	. . .	Recovered.	. . . .	
169	Côme.			F.	. . .	Recovered.	. . . .	
170	Côme.			F.	. . .	Died.	. . . .	
171	Côme.			M.	. . .	Died.	. . . .	
172	Côme.			M.	. . .	Died.	. . . .	"
173	Côme.			M.	. . .	Recovered.	. . . .	"
174	Côme.			M.	. . .	Recovered.	. . . .	"
175	Côme.			M.	. . .	Recovered	. . . .	"
176	Côme.			M.	. . .	Recovered.	. . . .	"
177	Côme.			M.	. . .	Recovered.	. . . .	"
178	Côme.			M.	. . .	Recovered.	. . . .	"
179	Côme.			M.	. . .	Recovered.	. . . .	"
180	Côme.			M.	. . .	Recovered.	. . . .	"
181	Côme.			M.	. . .	Recovered.	. . . .	"
182	Côme.			M.	. . .	Recovered.	. . . .	"
183	Côme.			M.	. . .	Recovered.	. . . .	"
184	Le Blanc.	1773	Child	M.	. . .	Recovered.	. . . .	Belmas, p. 11. Günther, p. 306.
185	Baseilhac.	1784	18	F.	℥v.	Recovered.	. . . .	Belmas, p. 12. Humphrey, p. 105. Carpue, p. 163.
186	Lassus.	1736	6	F.	. . .	Recovered.	Perineal operation attempted.	Belmas, p. 12. Cooper, p. 137. Carpue, p. 166. Humphrey, p. 105.
187	Deschamp.	1786	6	M.	. . .	Recovered.		
188	Lauverjat.	1790	Adult	F.	. . .	Recovered.	. . . .	Günther, p. 306; pp. 33-35.
189	Fourcroy.	1792			. . .	Died.	30 hours after.	Günther, p. 306; also Der Hohe Steinschnitt.
190	Fourcroy.	1792			. . .	Died.		
191	Souberbeille.	1796	32	F.	℥i. ss.	Recovered	. . . .	Belmas, p. 87.
192	Souberbeille.	1800	72	F.	℥ii.	Recovered.	. . . .	" p. 93.
193	Souberbeille.	1809	16	F.	℥vi. ss.	Recovered.	. . . .	" p. 86.
194	Souberbeille.	1812	23	F.	℥v.	Recovered.	. . . .	" p. 86.

Date column (rows 167–183): Operated upon between 1780 and the date of the death of Frère Côme.

	NAME.	DATE.	AGE.	SEX.	SIZE.	RESULT.	OBSERVATIONS.	REFERENCES.
195	Souberbeille.	1813	64	M.	Chestnut.	Died.	Gangrene of lungs on the 46th day; lateral lithotomy 10 months prior; two stones removed.	Belmas, p. 139.
196	Souberbeille.	1817	64	M.	Turkey's egg.	Recovered.	. . . .	" p. 131.
197	Souberbeille.	1817	82	M.	Large.	Died.	Pleuritic effusion; suppuration of right lung.	" p. 83.
198	Souberbeille.	1817	63	M.	Several stones.	Recovered.	. . . .	" p. 103.
199	Souberbeille.	1817	75	M.	Pigeon's egg.	Recovered.	. . . .	" p. 98.
200	Souberbeille.	1817	77	M.	Egg.	Recovered.	. . . .	" p. 100.
201	Souberbeille.	1817	. .	M.	Hen's egg.	Recovered.	. . . .	" p. 245.
202	Souberbeille.	1818	58	M.	Hen's egg.	Recovered.	. . . .	" p. 299.
203	Souberbeille.	1818	73	M.	. . .	Recovered.	. . . .	" p. 157.
204	Souberbeille.	1818	15	M.	℥iij.	Died.	Fungoid growth of prostate filled the bladder; kidney much diseased.	" p. 298.
205	Souberbeille.	1818	Adult	M.	7 oval calculi.	Recovered.	. . . .	" p. 136.
206	Souberbeille.	1818	73	M.	℥iij.	Died.	Enteritis; stone in both kidneys; scrofulous patient.	" p. 282.
207	Souberbeille.	1818	55	M.	5 small calculi.	Recovered.	. . . .	" p. 136.
208	Souberbeille.	1818	15	M.	Large.	Died.	Kidney disease.	" p. 294.
209	Souberbeille.	1818	60	M.	15 small calculi.	Died.	Enlarged kidneys; pyelitis; bladder contracted; diarrhœa.	" p. 109.
210	Souberbeille.	1818	68	M.	3 stones.	Died.	. . . .	" p. 292.
211	Souberbeille.	1818	69	M.	Large almond.	Recovered.	. . . .	" p. 280.
212	Souberbeille.	1818	64	M.	2 chestnuts.	Recovered.	Lateral, failed.	" p. 142.
213	Souberbeille.	1818	66	M.	Large hen's egg.	Died.	Lateral, 6 years previous; kidney contained many stones.	" p. 288.
214	Souberbeille.	1820	3¾	M.	Almond.	Recovered.	Although in a very bad condition from dentition and the effects of the stone.	" p. 216.
215	Souberbeille.	1821	58	F.	Walnut.	Recovered.	. . . .	" p. 277.
216	Souberbeille.	1822	54	M.	Hen's egg.	Died.	Peritonitis.	" p. 288.
217	Souberbeille.	1823	74	M.	3 large.	Died.	Pleuro-pneumonia.	" p. 297.
218	Souberbeille.	1823	63	M.	2 stones.	Recovered.	. . . .	" p. 160.

	NAME.	DATE.	AGE.	SEX.	SIZE.	RESULT.	OBSERVATIONS.	REFERENCES.
219	Souberbeille.	1823	70	M.	3 walnuts.	Died.	Acute nephritis; kidneys filled with pus.	Belmas, p. 88.
220	Souberbeille.	1823	58	M.	1, walnut; another size of a goose egg.	Died.	. . . .	" p. 158.
221	Souberbeille.	1823	70	M.	3 stones.	Recovered.	. . . .	" p. 138.
222	Souberbeille.	1824	40	M.	℥vss.	Recovered.	. . . .	" p. 134.
223	Souberbeille.	1824	71	M.	Large number of fragments equal in volume to hen's egg.	Recovered.	. . . .	" p. 135.
224	Souberbeille.	1824	66	M.	3 stones in all, equal to hen's egg.	Died.	7th day.	" p. 211.
225	Souberbeille.	1825	70	M.	2 stones; one the size of small hen's egg, the other smaller.	Died.	. . . .	" p. 120.
226	Souberbeille.	1824	58	M.	Hen's egg.	Recovered.	. . . .	" p. 287.
227	Souberbeille.	1825	31	M.	Very large; removed fragments.	Died.	59 days after; cancer of bladder, left kidney enlarged, filled with pus; also enteritis.	" p. 152.
228	Souberbeille.	1825	48	M.	Macaroon.	Recovered.	. . . .	" p. 287.
229	Souberbeille.	1825	68	M.	Large almond.	Recovered.	. . . .	" p. 300.
230	Souberbeille.	1825	74	M.	10 stones, equal to ℥i. gr. ii.	Recovered.	. . . .	" p. 150.
231	Souberbeille.	1825	74	M.	2 stones.	Recovered.	. . . .	" p. 275.
232	Souberbeille.	1825	74	M.	12 stones, size of chestnuts.	Died.	Apoplexy.	" p. 151.
233	Souberbeille.	1825	45	M.	Turkey's egg.	Died.	Kidneys enlarged; the pelvis of each contained stones; wound did not heal; patient was in a very bad state before operation.	" p. 106.
234	Souberbeille.	1825	83	M.	Hen's egg.	Died.	Gastro-enteritis.	" p. 291.
235	Souberbeille.	1826	62	M.	℥iv.	Died.	Kidneys much enlarged; ureters dilated and filled with purulent material; some urinary infiltration; was in a very bad condition before the operation.	" p. 278.
236	Souberbeille.	1826	67	M.	4 Walnut-size; 1 smaller.	Died.	Pneumonia.	" p. 235.

	NAME.	DATE.	AGE.	SEX.	SIZE.	RESULT.	OBSERVATIONS.	REFERENCES.
237	Souberbeille.	1826	62	M.	20 small, size of hazelnuts.	Recovered.	. . . .	Belmas, p. 23.
238	Souberbeille.	1826	70	M.	4, size of almonds.	Died.	Pneumonia.	" p. 234.
239	Souberbeille.	1826	74	M.	7, size of hazelnuts.	Recovered.	. . . .	" p. 235.
240	Souberbeille.	1826	8	M.	. . .	Recovered.	. . . .	" p. 237.
241	Souberbeille.	1826	75	M.	Almond.	Recovered.	. . . .	" p. 238.
242	Souberbeille.	1826	47	M.	℥vss.	Recovered.	. . . .	" p. 240.
243	Souberbeille.	1826	68	M.	Horse-chestnut.	Recovered.	. . . .	" p. 241.
244	Souberbeille.	1828	78	M.	300 calculi, equal in weight to ℥iii. or ℥iv.	Died.	Apoplexy. The stones were lodged in the folds of the bladder, thus making their extraction very tedious; there were 2 inguinal and 1 umbilical hernia.	The cases from No. 244 to 282 inclusive, are from the Mémoire de l'Académie Roy. de Méd., pp. 57 to 77; also p. 97, year 1840.
245	Souberbeille.	1828	70	M.	Chestnut.	Died.	. . . .	"
246	Souberbeille.	1828	72	M.	Chestnut.	Recovered.	. . . .	"
247	Souberbeille.	1829	71	M.	℥ii. ℨiii.	Recovered.	. . . .	"
248	Souberbeille.	1829	80	M.	℥ii.	Recovered.	. . . .	"
249	Souberbeille.	1829	66	M.	℥iv. ℨvi.	Recovered.	. . . .	"
250	Souberbeille.	1829	63	M.	℥vi.	Died.	Exhaustion.	"
251	Souberbeille.	1829	18	M.	℥i.	Recovered.	. . . .	"
252	Souberbeille.	1829	52	M.	℥ii. ℨvi.	Recovered.	. . . .	"
253	Souberbeille.	1829	21	M.	. . .	Died.	Peritonitis.	"
254	Souberbeille.	1829	65	M.	℥v.	Died.	Diphtheria.	"
255	Souberbeille.	1829	73	M.	℥ii.	Died.	Meteorism.	"
256	Souberbeille.	1829	70	M.	℥iv. ℨii.; 2 stones.	Recovered.	. . . .	"
257	Souberbeille.	1829	65	M.	℥v. ℨi.	Recovered.	. . . .	"
258	Souberbeille.	1830	75	M.	4 stones.	Recovered.	. . . .	"
259	Souberbeille.	1830	65	M.	℥iiss.	Recovered.	. . . .	"
260	Souberbeille.	1830	77	M.	℥iiss.	Recovered.	. . . .	"
261	Souberbeille.	1830	68	M.	3 stones.	Recovered.	. . . .	"
262	Souberbeille.	1830	73	M.	. . .	Recovered.	. . . .	"
263	Souberbeille.	1830	42	F.	℥iv.	Recovered.	. . . .	"
264	Souberbeille.	1830	54	M.	℥iv.	Died.	Peritoneum wounded; kidneys diseased; bladder scirrhous, etc	"

	NAME.	DATE.	AGE.	SEX.	SIZE.	RESULT.	OBSERVATIONS.	REFERENCES.
265	Souberbeille.	1830	65	M.	℥iii.	Died.	Hemorrhage, source of blood not clear.	Mémoire de l'Académie Roy. de Méd., 1840.
266	Souberbeille.	1830	68	M.	. . .	Died.	Exhaustion.	"
267	Souberbeille.	1830	59	M.	. . .	Recovered.	. . . .	"
268	Souberbeille.	1831	76	M.	℥iii.	Recovered.	. . . .	"
269	Souberbeille.	1831	72	M.	℥iv.	Died.	Typhoid fever.	"
270	Souberbeille.	1831	70	M.	3 stones.	Recovered.	. . . .	"
271	Souberbeille.	1832	70	M.	Egg.	Recovered.	. . . .	"
272	Souberbeille.	1832	67	M.	12 stones.	Recovered.	. . . .	"
273	Souberbeille.	1832	78	M.	℥iss.	Recovered.	. . . .	"
274	Souberbeille.	1833	63	M.	℥ii.	Recovered.	. . . .	"
275	Souberbeille.	1833	62	M.	℥ii.	Recovered.	. . . .	"
276	Souberbeille.	1833	64	M.	℥i. ℥ii.	Recovered.	. . . .	"
277	Souberbeille.	1833	69	M.	℥ii. ℥ss.	Recovered.	. . . .	"
278	Souberbeille.	1833	80	M.	2 stones.	Recovered.	. . . .	"
279	Souberbeille.	1833	74	M.	5 stones.	Died.	Urethro-rectal abscess.	"
280	Souberbeille.	1833	55	M.	℥viii. ℥iiss.	Recovered.	. . . .	"
281	Souberbeille.	1834	70	M.	4 stones.	Recovered.	. . . .	"
282	Souberbeille.	1834	54	M.	2 stones.	Recovered.	. . . .	"
283	Mursinna.	1797	30	M.	. . .	Died.	Phthisis; no sound could be passed; obstinate stricture of urethra, and on 5th day, asthenia.	Günther, p. 306.
284	Dupuytren.	1802	62	M.	℥viii.	Recovered.	. . . .	Belmas, p. 12. Hemphrey, p. 105. Lon. Med. Gaz., vol. i, p. 367. Archiv. für Klin. Chir., 1881, p. 54.
285	Scarpa.	1808	. .	F.	. . .	Recovered	. . . .	Belmas, p. 13. Günther, p. 306.
286	Vacca Berlinghieri.	1808	72	F.	. . .	Recovered.		
287	Berlinghieri.	1809	2	M.	. . .	Recovered.		
288	Berlinghieri.		25	M.	. . .	Died.	Peritonitis and urinary infiltration.	Günther, pp. 306 and 303.
289	Berlinghieri.		. .	. .	℥iii.	Died.	Urinary infiltration.	"
290	Berlinghieri.	1812 to 1816	. .	. .	. . .	Died.	Abscess and several calculi.	"
291	Berlinghieri.		. .	. .	. . .	Died.	. . . .	"

	NAME.	DATE.	AGE.	SEX.	SIZE.	RESULT.	OBSERVATIONS.	REFERENCES.
292	Unknown.	1811	28	F.	. . .	Died.	Removed an "etui," 21st day.	Poulet, vol. ii, p. 235.
293	Kirby.	1818	40	M.	. . .	Recovered.	Removed an elastic catheter.	Günther, pp. 306 and 334. Kirby's cases, p. 92. Belmas, p. 13. Cooper, vol. iii, p. 139. Humphrey, p. 103.
294	Home.	1820	16	M.	ʒi.	Recovered.	. . . .	Günther, pp. 44 and 45, in Der Hohe Steinschnitt,
295	Home.	1820	Child.	M.	. . .	Recovered.	. . . .	refers to all three cases but the following ref-
296	Home.	1820	Adult	U.	. . .	Recovered.	. . . .	erences: Archiv der Med., vol. i, p. 142. Belmas, p. 13. Humphrey, p. 105. Carpue, p. 167. Cooper, p. 207, refers to the 1st case only.
297	Delpech.	1820	. .	. .	. . .	Died.	48th day.	Günther, p. 335.
298	A German sur- geon.	1820	. .	. .	. . .	Recovered.	. . . .	Belmas, p. 13.
299	Dzondi.	1822	30	M.	. . .	Died.	. . . .	
300	Dzondi.	1822	30	M.	. . .	Recovered.	. . . .	
301	Dzondi.	1823	53	M.	. . .	Recovered.	. . . .	Günther, p. 335.
302	Dzondi.	1823	30	M.	. . .	Recovered.	. . . .	
303	Deguise.	1822	30	M.	ʒxxxi.	Died.	. . . .	
304	Hutchinson.	1824	73	M.	. . .	Died.	This operation was for the removal of a large clot of blood follow- ing hemorrhage, and from a fungoid tu- mor of the prostate.	Günther, p. 46, in Der Hohe Steinschnitt. Lond. Med. Gaz., New Series, vol. xxii, p. 12. Anderson, Quart. Med. Science, 1824–6, p. 134, vol. iii. Edin. Med. & Surg. Jour- nal, vol. xxvii, p. 188.
305	Hutchinson.	1825	20	M.	2 inches in di- ameter, and 1½ broad.	Recovered.	. . . .	Lond. Med. Repos., New Series, vol. i, p. 559. Günther, p. 306. Cooper, vol. ii, p. 267.
306	Ballingall.	1826	. .	. .	. . .	Died.	Operation not finished.	Humphrey, p. 105. Günther, p. 306.
307	Ewbank.	1827 (about.)	. .	. .	. . .	Died.	. . . .	Humphrey, p. 100.
308	Krimer.	1827	23	. .	ʒxxiii.	Recovered.	. . . .	Velpeau, vol. iii, p. 960. Cooper, vol. ii, p. 209.
309	Roux.	1827	Very old.	M.	. . .	Died.	15th day, urinary infil- tration and abscess.	Günther, p. 306. Humphrey, p. 105. Velpeau, vol. iii, p. 960. Cooper, p. 137.
310	Amussat.	1827	65	M.	. . .	Recovered.		

NAME.	DATE.	AGE.	SEX.	SIZE.	RESULT.	OBSERVATIONS.	REFERENCES.
311 Amussat.	1827	69	M.	. . .	Recovered	. . . .	Günther, in Der Hohe Steinschnitt, pp. 49-52.
312 Amussat.	1827	76	M.	. . .	Recovered.		
313 Amussat.	1827	2½	M.	. . .	Recovered.		
314 Amussat.	1827	4	M.	. . .	Recovered.		
315 Amussat.	1834	12	M.	. . .	Recovered.		
316 Amussat.	1834	67	M.	. . .	Died.	Infiltration of urine.	Le Courrier Méd., July 15, 1876.
317 Crozat.	1828	. .	F.	. . .	Recovered.	Peritoneum was laid open to a considerable extént.	Velpeau, vol. iii, p. 966.
318 Baudens.	1829	23	M.	. . .	Recovered.	. . . .	
319 Baudens.	1829	6	M.	. . .	Recovered.	. . . .	Report Hop. du Midi, 1830, p. 290-2. Sabattier, vol. iv, p. 249. Günther, p. 306.
320 Baudens.	1829	5½	M.	. . .	Recovered.		
321 Lisfranc.	1829	. .	. .	℥vii.	Recovered.		
322 Lisfranc.	1829	. .	. .	. . .	Died.	Infiltration of urine.	Lond. Med. Gaz., 1829, vol. v, p. 123.
323 Lisfranc.	. . .	. .	. .	. . .	Died.	Infiltration of urine.	Lond. Med. Gaz., 1829, vol. v, p. 123.
324 Bell.	1829	80	. .	. . .	Recovered.	. . . .	London Lancet, 1833, p. 668.
325 Catereau.	1832	57	F.	Very large.	Recovered.	. . . .	Gaz. Med., 1832, p. 777.
326 Rognette.	1833	44	M.	Small walnut.	Recovered.	. . . .	Gaz. Med., 1836, p. 373. Velpeau, vol. iii, p. 960.
327 Voisson.	1834	56	M.	. . .	Died.	Gangrene 3d day; stone not wholly removed; a portion remaining strangulated behind the prostate.	
328 Voisson.	1839	35	M.	. . .	Recovered.		
329 Leroy d'Etiolles.	1834	70	M.	. . .	Died.	8th day, stone encysted; not removed; pelvic cellulitis.	Günther, pp. 306 and 335.
330 Seger.	1835 to 1846	5	M.	. . .	Recovered.	. . . .	Günther. Der Hohe Steinschnitt, p. 306.
331 Seger.		27	M.	. . .	Recovered.		
332 Seger.		8	M.	. . .	Recovered.		
333 Cazeneuve.	1836	9	M.	. . .	Died.	47 hours after peritonitis.	Mémoire Acad. Roy, 1837, p. 407.
334 Rufz.	1836	49	M.	. . .	Recovered.	. . . .	Gaz. Med., 1839, p. 509.

NAME.	DATE.	AGE.	SEX.	SIZE.	RESULT.	OBSERVATIONS.	REFERENCES.
335 Bancal.	1838	58	M.	. . .	Died.	. . . .	Bancal, p. 119.
336 Tonnellé.	1839	..	..	. . .	Died.	Hemorrhage.	Velpeau, vol. iii, p. 964.
337 Leonadon.	1839	..	..	. . .	Recovered.	. . . .	Velpeau, vol. iii, p. 960. Gaz. Med., 1839, p. 795.
338 Moulinié.	1839	Child.	M.	. . .	Died.	Obstinate stricture of urethra; bilateral first tried; stone was not removed.	Günther, p. 306.
339 Civiale.		..	..	. . .	Died.	. . . .	Günther, p. 306.
340 Civiale.	1841 to 1844	..	..	. . .	Recovered.	. . . .	" "
341 Civiale.		..	..	. . .	Recovered.	. . . .	" "
342 Civiale.		..	..	. .· .	Recovered.	. . . .	" "
343 Civiale.		..	..	. . .	Recovered.	. . . .	" "
344 Larrey.	1841	33	F.	. . .	Recovered.	. . . .	" "
345 Smith.	1841	30	M.	ʒi. ʒii. gr. viii.	Died.	Phthisis; exhaustion.	Günther, p. 306; Lancet, April, 1841, p. 118.
346 Nelaton.	1841	73	M.	15, each size of apricot-stone.	Died.	9th day, exhaustion.	Gunther, p. 306.
347 Segalas.	1844	37	M.	. . .	Recovered.	. . . .	Gaz. Med., 1844, p. 630.
348 Günther.	1845	29	M.	. . .	Recovered.		
349 Günther.	1845	Child.	..	. . .	Recovered.		
350 Günther.	1847	13	M.	. . .	Recovered.		
351 Günther.	1851	9	M.	. . .	Recovered.	. . . .	Günther, p. 335.
352 Günther.	1851	..	..	. . .	Recovered.		
353 Günther.	1851	..	..	. . .	Recovered.		
354 Günther.	1851 About.	..	..	. . .	Recovered.		
355 Günther.	1860	..	..	. . .	Recovered.		
356 Olivarez.	1848	..	..	. . .	Recovered.	. . . .	Günther, pp. 59 and 60, Der Hohe Steinschnitt.
357 Olivarez.	1848	..	..	. . .	Recovered.		
358 Olivarez.	1848	..	..	. . .	Recovered.		
359 Humphrey.	1848	14	M.	ʒi. ʒiv.	Recovered.	. . . .	Humphrey, p. 105.
360 Brüns.	1848	26	M.	. . .	Recovered.		
361 Brüns.	1848	17	M.	. . .	Recovered.	. . . .	Günther, p. 306.
362 Brüns.	1848	3	M.	. . .	Recovered.	. . . .	" "
363 Landouzy.	1848	Adult	M.	. . .	Recovered.	. . . .	Gaz. Med., 1849, p. 239.
364 Langenbeck.	1849	3½	..	. . .	Recovered.		

NAME.	DATE.	AGE.	SEX.	SIZE.	RESULT.	OBSERVATIONS.	REFERENCES.
365 Langenbeck.	. . .	. .	. .	. . .	Recovered.	. . . .	
366 Langenbeck.	. . .	. .	. .	. . .	Recovered.	. . . .	
367 Langenbeck.	. . .	. .	. .	. . .	Recovered.	. . . .	Günther, p. 306.
368 Langenbeck.	. . .	. .	. .	. . .	Died.	3d day.	Deutsch. Klin., 1850.
369 Schlobig.	1850	15	M.	. . .	Died.	Pleuro-pneumonia; ulceration above pubes; gangrene.	Günther, p. 306.
370 Unger.	1850	2¾	M.	. . .	Died.	. . . .	Günther, p. 306.
371 Geinitz.	1851	27	U.	. . .	Died.	4 days, uræmia; left kidney atrophied; right, hypertrophied.	Günther, p. 306.
372 Huguier.	1852	34	M.	. . .	Died.	. . . .	Bulletin de la Soc. de Chir., 1852, p. 306.
373 Staude.	1854	. .	. .	. . .	Recovered.		
374 Staude.	. . .	. .	. .	. . .	Recovered.		
375 Staude.	. . .	. .	. .	. . .	Recovered.	. . . .	Günther, p. 335.
376 Staude.	. . .	. .	. .	. . .	Recovered.		
377 D'Almeida. This surgeon operated on 22 cases; 7 died and the remainder were all successful. . . . . . . The particulars of these cases have not been found.	1860 . . .	30 . .	M. . .	. . . . . .	Recovered. 7 died, 16 recovered.	. . . .	Dict. Encyc. des Science Med., vol. xxv, part 1st, p. 103.
400 Vitellius.	. . .	. .	. .	ʒxxii.	Recovered.	. . . .	Archiv für Klin. Chir., 1881, p. 48.
401 Uytterhoeven.	. . .	. .	. .	ʒxlii.	Died.	9th day.	Archiv für Klin. Chir., 1881, p. 48.
402 Von Graefe.	. . .	. .	M.	ʒxxiss.	Recovered.	. . . .	Erichsen, vol. ii, p. 772. Coulson, p. 476.
403 Hahn.	. . .	46	F.	. . .	Died.	Hair-pin was the nucleus of the stone; had been in the bladder for 30 years. Up to the 14th day after the operation she had no fever, when she suddenly died of uræmia; she had hydronephrosis; one ureter was entirely obliterated, the other partly so.	Archiv für Klin. Chir., 1881, p. 53.
404 Stilling.	. . .	58	M.	. . .	Recovered.	. . . .	Archiv für Klin. Chir., 1881, p. 53.
405 Gamgee.	1861	8	F.	. . .	Recovered.	. . . .	Lancet, vol. ii, 1873, p. 807.

NAME.	DATE.	AGE.	SEX.	SIZE.	RESULT.	OBSERVATIONS.	REFERENCES.
406 Chisholm.	1862	Adult	M.	. . .	Recovered.	Shot above the pelvis; bullet lodged in the bladder by the operation.	Med. and Surg. History of the Rebellion, part ii, vol. ii, p. 282.
407 McGill.	1862	Adult	M.	. . .	Died.	Shot above the pubis; lodged in bladder.	Same as above.
408 Hammer.	1865	1½	. .	. . .	Died.	18 hours after, of convulsions, following a bath.	St. Louis Med. and Surg. Journ., p. 51.
409 Dever.	1867	9¼	M.	. . .	Recovered.	. . . .	Bulletin de Thérapeutique, vol. 92, p. 13.
410 Dever.	1869	9	M.	. . .	Recovered.		
411 Simon.	1867 About.	6	M.	. . .	Died.	Erysipelas.	Deutsch. Klin., 1867, p. 23.
412 Mercier.	1867	54	M.	. . .	Recovered.	. . . .	Mercier, p. 456.
413 Adams.	1868	Adult	M.	. . .	Recovered.	Failure after lateral.	Med. Times and Gazette, Oct. 16, 1878.
414 Amussat fils.	1876	2	M.	. . .	Recovered.	. . .	Le Courrier Méd., July, 1876, p. 219.
415 Amussat fils.	1876	16	M.	. . .	Recovered.		
416 Trendelenberg.	1877	2	M.	. . .	Recovered.	. . . .	Lond. Med. Rec., Feb. 15, 1877. Berlin Klin. Wöch, Mar. 2, 1877.
417 Fowler.	1877	16	M.	. . .	Recovered.	After failure of lithotrity and lateral lithotomy.	Monthly Abs. Med. Science, Dec., 1878.
418 Keyes.	1877	75	M.	. . .	Died.	In very low condition before operation; the others were in the same desperate state.	Medical Record, 1877, p. 234.
419 Keyes.	1877	73	M.	. . .	Died.	"	
420 Keyes.	1877	65	M.	. . .	Died.	"	
421 Helmuth.	1878	53	M.	℥iij. Ʒjss.	Recovered.		Vide page 65.
422 Helmuth.	1878	70	M.	℥iij. grs. x.	Died.	Shock.	" " 69.
423 Helmuth.	1879	65	M.	3 calculi. ℥iss. grs. xii.	Died.	Gangrene of bladder; in very bad condition at time of operation.	" " 72.
424 Helmuth.	1882	70	M.	℥j. Ʒij. Ʒj.	Recovered.	Failure of litholapaxy.	" " 73.
425 Rachel.	1878	5	M.	gr. xliv.	Recovered.	. . . .	Am. Journ. Med. Sciences, 1879, p. 117.
426 J. Hutchinson.	1878	26	M.	℥viss.	Died.	Pyæmia 5 weeks after.	Med. Times and Gazette, Oct. 19, 1878.
427 Leschick.	1878	5	M.	4 inches long, 9 inches circumference.	Recovered.	18 days in healing; patient was made to lie on the stomach for the first five days.	Berlin Klin. Wöch, 4th Mars, 1872.
428 Doughty.	1880	39	M.	℥iij. Ʒij. grs. xxx	Recovered.	Failure of litholapaxy.	
429 Billroth.	1880	30	M.	. . .	Died.	Phthisical patient; exhaustion.	
430 Groves.	1880	30	M.	6 cal., 5 an inch in diameter, 6th smaller.	Recovered.	. . . .	Canadian Journ. Med. Sc., Nov. 1881, p. 354.
431 Groves.	1880	6	M.	. . .	Recovered.		

SUPRAPUBIC LITHOTOMY.

TABLE A.*

Dr. Dulles's Table of Suprapubic Lithotomies performed by American Surgeons only.

No.	Surgeon	Date	Age of patient	Sex	Size or weight of calculus	Recovered	Died	Time after operation in days	Reference	Remarks
1	Gibson.	1824	Old.	M.	2 calculi.	...	D.	....	Gibson's Surgery, 1835.	Was doing very well, but withdrew his catheter, and peritonitis set in.
2	Carpenter.	1827	8	M.	2 "	R.	...	....	Am. Med. Rec., No. 39, 1827, p. 199; Eclectic Med. Journ. of Medicine, vol. ii, May, 1838, p 288.	
3	McClellan.	...	....	...		R	...		Gross, Diseases of Urinary Organs, p. 632.	
4	McClellan.	...	......	...		R.	...		" " "	
5	McClellan.	...	......	...		R.	...		" " "	
6	McClellan.	..	.....	..			D.		" " "	
7	McClellan.	...							" " "	Constitution very much shattered by previous disease.
8	Gardner.	1844	42	M.	℥ixss.	R.	..	......	Gross, Kentucky Surgery, p. 105; Letter of Gardner, Feb. 16, 1875.	Immediately after *failure of perineal operation.*
9	W. L. Atlee.	1848	Man.	M.	Circumference 4".	R.	...	....	Eve, Remarkable Cases in Surgery.	*Lateral operation had failed six months before.*
10	De Valetti.	1849	"	M.	℥iv.	R.	...	38	New Orleans Med. and Surg. Journ., Sept. 1849, p. 176.	Calculus 18 years.
11	Delery.	1850	12	M.	℥ix.	R.	...	30	L'Union Médicale de Louisiana, No. 3, March, 1852, p. 46.	Applied sulph. of iron and camphor to prevent urinary infiltration.
12	Pope.	1850	22	M.	℥iij. ℥vss., and as much more.	...	D.	3	St. Louis Med. and Surgical Journal, Sept. and Oct., 1864	*Did perineal operation also,* and tunnelled through and through the calculus.
13	W. J. Johnson.	1851	18	M.	℥vj.	...	D.	4	Southern Med. Journ., Dec., 1851, p. 727.	*Perineal operation had failed,* and also a great many ineffectual attempts to crush.
14	Parker.	1853	33	F.	2" / 1½".	R.	...	....	N. Y. Med. Journ., Mar., 1855, p. 252.	
15	Parker.	1853	53	F.	....	R.	...	......	" " "	
16	Parker.	1854	47	F.	....	R.	...	......	" " "	
17	Parker.	1855	62	F.	....	R.	...		Letter of Dr. Parker, Sept. 21, '74.	
18	Parker.	1857	53	M		...	D.	4	Letter of Dr. Parker, Sept. 21, 1874, and also Am. Med. Times, July 7, 1860.	Died of emesis from inflammation of stomach.
19	Pitcher.	1854	8	F.	℥iij.	R.	...	......	Letter of Dr. S. H. Douglas, Oct. 5, 1874.	
20	Eve.	1855	66	M	℥j. ℥ij	R.	...	18	Trans. Am. Med. Association, '71, vol. xxii, p. 273.	
21	Eve.	1858	28	M.	℥iv. ℥ij.	...	D.	3		Peritonitis.
22	Weber.	1856	4	F.		R.	...	12	N. Y. Med. Journ., July, 1856, p. 45.	
23	Noeggerath.	1857	8	M.	℥ij.	R.	...	25	N. Y. Med. Journ., Jan., 1858, p. 9.	
24	Hewitt.	1859	19	M.	....	R.	...	21	N. Y. Med. Journ., Mar., 1859, p. 217.	
25	Krackowizer.	1859	1½	M.	....	...*	D.	1	Am. Med. Times, July 7, 1860	Died of emesis from chloroform.
26	Krackowizer.	1860	3	M.			D.	......	" " "	Died of pneumonia.
27	Krackowizer.	...	Boy.	M.			D.	2	" " "	
28	Krackowizer.	...	"	M			D.		Letter of Dr. K., Sept. 23, 1874.	
29	Krackowizer.	..	"	M.		R.				
30	Krackowizer.	..	"	M.		R				
31	Wood.	1860	58	M.	Pigeon'segg	...	D.	2	Am. Med. Times, July 7, 1860.	Peritoneum cut in two places.
32	Felton.	1862	....	M.		...	D.	1	Nashville Journ. of Med. and Surg., Jan., 1867, p. 502.	To remove a shrapnel shot.
33	Mackenzie.	.	2½			R.	...		Letter from Dr. M., Aug. 29, 1874.	
34	Westmoreland.	1863	7	F.		R.	...	..	Letter from Dr. C. H. Mastin, Jan. 1, 1875.	
35	Robertson.	1865	56	M.	℥j. ℥vj.	R	...	35	Pacific Med. and Surg. Journ., April, 1868, p 499.	Placed in a semi-sitting posture for 48 hours after operation.
36	Guido Bell.	1867	4½	M.	grs. xvj.	R.	...	26	Memorabilien Heilbronn, Mar. 28, 1874, p. 552.	Bladder sewed up; catheter pulled out same evening.
37	Guido Bell.	1872	3	M.	℥jss.	R.	.	21		Peritoneum cut, but no harm resulted.
38	Bock.	1873	6	M.	℥j	R.	...	21	Letter of Dr. B., Sept. 10, 1874.	
39	Bock.	1874	3	M.		R.	...		Letter of Dr. B., Dec. 8, 1874.	
40	H. Lenox Hodge	1874	52	M.	℥jss.	...	D.	2	C. W. D.	Immediately after *failure of perineal operation.*
41	Edw. Geddings	1856	8	M.	2½ long.	...	D.	10	Letter of Dr. G., May 13, 1875.	
42	Bailey.	1874	2½		54 grs.	R.	...	25	Letter of Dr. B., May 28, 1875.	
43	Eli Geddings.	1874	40	M.	....	R.	...		Letter from Dr. G., May 13, '75.	

* American Journal of the Medical Sciences, January, 1875.

TABLE B.*

Suprapubic Lithotomies, from 1867 to 1877.—(Dr. Dulles.)

SURGEON.	DATE.	AGE.	DESCRIPTION OF CALCULI.	RESULT.	TIME AFTER OPERATION OF RECOVERY OR DEATH.	REFERENCES.
Mercier.	1867	30	℥ij. ℥iiiss.	R.	46 days.	Gazette Hebdom., 1869, p. 583.
Bell.	1867	4½	grs. xvi.	R.	26 "	Western Journ. of Med., Nov., 1867.
Bell.	1872	3	grs. xcvi.	R.	21 "	Memorabilien Heilbronn, March 28, 1874.
Bell.	1875	2	℥ij.	R.	30 "	Indiana Journ. of Med., Aug., 1875.
Bell.	1875	3½	Large bean size.	R.	62 "	Am. Practitioner, March, 1876.
Brodie.	1868	35	Walnut size.	R.	. . . .	Letter from Dr Brodie, May 5, 1876.
Brady.	1868	42	℥iss.	R.	21 "	Detroit Rec. of Med. Pharm., Sept., 1869.
Betz.	1869	6	Acorn size.	R.	42 "	Memorabilien Heilbronn, Feb. 28, 1874.
Betz.	1870	8	Cherry size.	R.	42 "	Memorabilien Heilbronn, Feb. 28, 1874.
Deering.	1870	46	2 { ℥iv. grs.xx. ℥v. grs.xiv.	R.	14 "	Med. and Surg. Rep., April 29, 1876.
Watson.	1871	56	℥viiiss.	R.	42 "	Letter from Dr. Watson, Oct. 6, 1874.
Bock.	1873	6	℥j.	R.	21 "	Letter from Dr. Bock, Sept. 10, 1874.
Bock.	1874	3	grs. xxv.	R.	12 "	Letter from Dr. Bock, Dec. 8, 1874.
Bock.	1874	4	grs. lvijss.	R.	11 "	Letter from Dr. Bock, Jan. 30, 1878.
Bailey.	1874	2½	grs. liv.	R.	21 "	Letter from Dr. Bailey, May 28, 1875.
Billroth.	1874	12	Tumor apple size.	R.	33 "	Letter from Dr. Karl Schwaighofer, Nov. 3, 1874.
Langenbeck.	1875	1¾	Date-seed size.	R.	35 "	Arch. f. Klin. Chir.-Bd., xxi, Sup. Heft., S. 210.
Rachel.	1875	4	℥ij.	D.	7 "	This article.
Starr.	1876	35	℥i. ℥i.	R.	16 "	Am. Journ. Med. Sciences, July, 1877.
Fletcher.	1876	2½	grs. lxiijss.	D.	2 "	Letter from Dr. Fletcher, Jan. 30, 1878.

Recovered, 18   Average time of recovery, 29 days.
Died,   2   Death ratio, 1 in 10.
Total,   20

* Tables A and B are taken from Dulles's articles; with these exceptions, all the other references have a carefully examined. American Journal of the Medical Sciences, April, 1878.

TABLE C.*

Operations in which the Result is Unknown.

	Date.	Reference.
A surgeon of Strasburg, . . .	1727.	Günther, page 306.
Hess, ...	1729.	" "
Kulmus, ...	1732.	" "
Le Cat, 3 cases, ...	1735.	" "
Anthelme, ...	1828.	" "
Josephi, ...	1828.	" "
Paully, 3 cases, ...	1843.	" "
Gaillard, ...	1844.	" "
Paine, ...	1848.	" "
Frenzel, ...	1848.	" "
Pech, ...	1848.	" "
Fleury, ...	1852.	" "
Stolle, ...	1856.	" "
Berger, ...	1856.	" "
Schmidt, ...	1856.	" "
Morlanne, ...	1856.	" "
Remmers, ...	. .	" "
Lotzbeck, ...	1858.	" "
Breslau, ...	. .	" "

Mandt, }
Noel, } Velpeau, vol. iii, pp. 948–964.

Lagouest, Archiv für Klin. Chir., 1880, vol. xxv.

Vollemeier, Gaz. Med., p. 240.

Billroth, 2 cases.

Petersen, 4 cases. Am. Journ. Med. Science, April, 1881, p. 573.

TABLE D.

A General Summary of the Operations since 1561.

Author.	Recovered.	Died.	Unknown. Result.	Total.
Rankin, ...	312	119	33	464
Dulles's 1st Table, ...	28	14	1	43
" 2d "	18	2	. .	20
Total, ...	358	135	34	527

* These cases are omitted from all the tables which follow.

TABLE E.

Operations performed since 1878.

No.	NAME.	DATE.	AGE.	SEX.	SIZE.	RESULT.	REMARKS.
1	Helmuth.	1878	53	M.	ʒiij. Əiss.	Recovered.	
2	Helmuth.	1878	70	M.	ʒiij. grs. x.	Died.	Shock.
3	Helmuth.	1879	65	M.	3 calculi. ʒiss. grs. xij.	Died.	Gangrene of bladder.
4	Helmuth.	1882	70	M.	ʒj. ʒij. Əj.	Recovered.	Much debility; failure of litholapaxy.
5	Rachel.	1878	5	M.	grs. xlv.	Recovered.	Am. Journ. Med. Sci., 1879, p. 117.
6	Hutchinson.	1878	26	M.	ʒvi. ss.	Died of Pyæmia.	Med. Times and Gazette, Oct. 19, 1878.
7	Leschick.	1878	5	M.	. . . . .	Recovered.	Berlin Klin. Woch., March 4, 1878.
8	Billroth.	1880	30	M.	. . . . .	Died.	
9	Doughty.	1880	39	M.	ʒiij. ʒij. grs. xxx.	Recovered.	Bigelow's litholapaxy failed.
10	Groves.	1881	67	M.	6 calculi; 5 about 1 inch diameter.	Recovered.	Canada Journal of Medical Sciences, Nov., 1881.
11	Groves.	1881	63	M.	. . . . .	Recovered.	

In statistical comparisons between different operations, the causes of death are, perhaps, the most important topic, and the discussion of this subject is the greatest benefit to be deduced from such a computation. The subject has been divided into two sections. The first including those causes which are due to the operation itself; the second into those which arose from sources independent of the operation.

A large number of cases (forty-two) have necessarily been omitted as being defective in this particular. In the other tables which follow, similar omissions have been made, thus giving a variety of figures, for in some instances there is no record of the sex, in others none of the age, and in others the date is deficient.

TABLE F.

Causes of Death arising from the Operation.

Abscess and sloughing of wound,	1
Peritonitis,	11
Peritonitis and urinary infiltration,	1
Pelvic cellulitis,	2
Hemorrhage,	5
Cystitis,	1
Blood poisoning,	1
Asthenia,	2
Wound of peritoneum,	2
Urinary infiltration,	5
Erysipelas,	1
Meteorism,	1
Gangrene of bladder, } " of wound, }	3
Shock,	1
Pyæmia,	3
	—
	40

TABLE G.

Causes of death NOT due to the Operation.

Suppuration of kidney with stone,	1
Convulsions,	2
Carcinoma of bladder,	4
Pyelitis,	3
Abscess of kidney,	2
Inflammation of kidney, with stone in the ureter,	1
Hydatids in pelvis of kidney,	1
Pleurisy,	2
Helminthiasis,	1
Gangrene of lung,	1
Asthenia from old age,	2
Disease of kidneys and stone,	5
Diarrhœa,	1
Pleuro-pneumonia,	2
Pneumonia,	3
Apoplexy,	2
Enteritis,	1
Gastro-enteritis,	1
Emesis from chloroform,	1
Gastritis,	1
Phthisis and phthisical exhaustion,	3
Urethro-rectal abscess,	1
Uræmia,	2
Unfinished operation ; non-removal of stone,	3
Debility from previous disease,	4
Diphtheria,	1
Acute nephritis,	1
Typhoid fever,	1
	—
	53
Causes not mentioned,	42
" from operation,	40
	—
	135

Thus it appears that 53 out of the 135 deaths cannot, with any fairness, be set down to the operation, and if these should be omitted from the general sum, together with those in whom the cause of death is not stated, we would have a remainder of 388 cases, with 40 deaths due to the method, giving a ratio of mortality as 1 in 9.7.

It is a curious coincidence that we obtain the same results in regard to the fatal cases as Dr. Dulles, whereas we differ materially in particulars. Dulles assigns only 25 accidents and complications as causes of death. He places pyæmia, phlebitis, and cystitis as not arising from the procedure, while " perineal operation complicating " " terrible operation," cannot be set down as very definite causes. These in this table have been set down as not stated.

The average size of the stones extracted by the suprapubic operation is exceptionally large. Among the largest are—Deguise's case, of ℥xxxi; Krimer's ℥xxiij; Vitellius's, ℥xxij; and Uytterhœven's, ℥xlij.

In those cases which have been adduced, the average weight of the calculus is about ℥ivss, whereas the average in the lateral method, according to the tables of Mr. Crosse, is between ℥i and ℥iss.

TABLE H.*

Showing the Results at Different Periods of Life as compared with the Lateral Method.

LATERAL.

AGES.	NO. OF CASES.	RECOVERED.	FATAL.	PROPORTION OF FATAL.	
1–10	734	688	46	1 in 15.73	Average age, 24.22 years.
10–20	298	266	32	1 in 9.31	
20–30	213	191	22	1 in 9.68	
30–40	164	134	30	1 in 5.46	
40–50	149	120	29	1 in 5.13	
50–60	182	143	39	1 in 4.66	
60–70	140	104	36	1 in 3.88	
70–80	28	18	10	1 in 2.80	
	1908	1664	244	1 in 7.81 $\frac{5}{8}\frac{9}{1}$	

* These cases are collected from the statistics of Cheselden, from the Williams table of the Norfolk and Norwich Hospital, and from those of the Saharunpore Dispensary.

SUPRAPUBIC.*

AGES.	No. of CASES.	RECOVERED.	FATAL.	PROPORTION OF FATAL.	
1–10	84	68	16	1 in 5.25	Average age, 32.83 years.
10–20	45	34	11	1 in 4.09	
20–30	29	23	6	1 in 4.83	
30–40	27	18	9	1 in 3.00	
40–50	23	19	4	1 in 5.75	
50–60	32	24	8	1 in 4.00	
60–70	52	34	18	1 in 2.88	
70–80	50	32	18	1 in 2.77	
	342	252	90	1 in 3.80	

In the lateral operations, assuming that all the cases under ten years average five, all between ten and twenty years, fifteen, all between twenty and thirty, twenty-five, all between thirty and forty, thirty-five, and so on, we obtain an average of 24.22 years.

There are 152 cases of suprapubic operation in which the age is not stated, leaving 342, the actual age of which is known, making an average of 32.82 fatal.

Thus it seems that the average age in the suprapubic operations is over 8 years more than that of the lateral. In 1908 cases of the latter, only 28 were over 70 years of age, whereas in 343 of the former, where the age is known, 50 had reached and passed that age. Again, 102 cases, or nearly one-third in the suprapubic operations, were over 60 years; in the lateral, only 168, or about one-eleventh. In glancing over the tables, the reader will see that Frère Côme and M. Souberbeille occupy a very prominent place; in fact, contributing together over one-third of the cases. It would only be natural, therefore, to ask for the results of these individually. Frère Côme, as has been stated, lost 19 in 100; but Souberbeille lost 31 out of 90, or a fraction over one-third. The cause of this great mortality, which at first glance seems to speak strongly against the operation, can in a great measure be explained as due, first, to the extreme age of his patients, several of whom were over 80 years of age; secondly, to the effects of previous disease. The average age of these cases is 61.92, or nearly 62 years. This extremely high average shows that the majority of these patients must have suffered from stone and numerous complications for years before submitting to the opera-

* This table includes 49 cases from Dr. Dulles's tables. The ages of the remainder of his cases are not stated.

tion. That this, is the case is well demonstrated by the fact that 22 out of the 31 deaths were due to causes, not from the operation. If these 22, together with 2 others in which the cause of death is not stated, should be omitted, M. Souberbeille's statistics would read, 66 operations with 7 deaths.

Thus, instead of the statistics arguing against this method, they show that the character of a large portion of cases has been of the most desperate and hopeless nature; and when these unfavorable conditions are set aside, and the operation put upon a fair basis and viewed from the same standpoint as the other methods, we find that the ratio of mortality compares favorably. (See table.)

TABLE I.

Table showing the Mortality in each Sex, compared with the Lateral Operation.

	LATERAL.*					SUPRAPUBIC.			
Sex.	Total.	Recovered.	Fatal.	Prop. Fatal.	Sex.	Total.	Recovered.	Fatal.	Prop. Fatal.
Males,	669	578	91	1 in 7.35	Males,	285	191	93	1 in 3.05
Females,	35	33	2	1 in 17.50	Females,	87	75	12	1 in 7.25
					Not stated,	122	92	30	

In the cases where the sex is not recorded it is very probable that the majority, if not all with a few exceptions, were "male." Assuming them as such, the figures would read: Total, 406; recovered, 283; died, 123; proportion fatal, 1 in 3.29.

TABLE K.

Showing the Mortality at Different Ages.

Ages.	Total.	Recovered.	Fatal.	Prop. Fatal.
Under 5,	41	34	7	1 in 5.85
5 to 10,	43	34	9	1 in 4.77
10 to 15,	21	16	5	1 in 4.20
15 to 20,	24	18	6	1 in 4.00
20 to 25,	13	11	2	1 in 6.50
25 to 30,	16	12	4	1 in 4.00
30 to 35,	17	10	7	1 in 2.42
35 to 40,	10	8	2	1 in 5.00
40 to 45,	11	11	0	1 in 0.00
45 to 50,	12	8	4	1 in 3.00
50 to 55,	12	10	2	1 in 6.00
55 to 60,	20	14	6	1 in 3.33
60 to 65,	25	20	5	1 in 5.00
65 to 70,	28	15	13	1 in 2.15
70 to 75,	33	18	15	1 in 2.20
75 to 80,	13	12	1	1 in 13.00
80 and over,	4	2	2	1 in 2.00
	343	253	90	

* From J. G. Crosse's "Treatise on Stone."

TABLE L.

Showing the General Results of Different Methods of Lithotomy.

	TOTAL.	RECOVERED.	FATAL.	PROP. FATAL.
Lateral . . .	10,150	9036	1114	1 in 9.11
Bilateral , . .	536	495	41	1 in 13.07
Median, . . .	350	318	32	1 in 10.93
Recto-vesical, .	83	67	16	1 in 5.18
Suprapubic, . .	493 or 388	358 or 348	135 or 40	1 in 3.65 or 1 in 9.70

* From Gross's " Diseases of the Bladder." p. 338.

CHAPTER III.

OPINIONS, OBJECTIONS, AND EXPERIMENTS RELATIVE TO SUPRAPUBIC
LITHOTOMY; THE ADVANTAGES OF THE OPERATION.

IT is quite curious, in reviewing the literature of this subject, to observe upon
what various grounds this operation has been considered unworthy of regard,
thus, an editor of the *Medico-Chirurgical Review*, in commenting upon Dr.
King's work,[*] gives the author's and his own opinion of the procedure in a
very few decisive words. He says, when speaking of the high operation : "As
Dr. King very justly observes, this operation is not only more liable than the
lateral operation to be succeeded by infiltration of urine into the cellular tissue,
but also by peritonitis, the two chief dangers of the latter. When we add
that the operation is *one of extreme difficulty, we pronounce its condemnation
in the most emphatic terms.* A very large stone has been supposed to be its
only justification, yet we venture to say, that if a calculus is too large to admit
of extraction by any operation but that above the pubes, *it were better not
extracted at all;* the patient must almost surely die." Mr. Holmes Coot has
stated the entire impossibility of the operation in many cases, and Lizars in his
Surgery, as also quoted by Dulles, says, "Sir Astley Cooper gives so horrible
a picture of an operator, in Paris, *wounding the peritonæum, and the intestines
protruding,* as to dissuade anyone from adopting this operation." It is just
such unfortunate expressions, written without any experience or any study of
the subject, which have, no doubt, deterred very many from attempting the
operation. The ideas promulgated in such texts are wrong. The operation is
not difficult, and is, as it has proved itself, particularly applicable to those cases
wherein the other methods have been unsuccessful, and with care there is but
little danger of wounding the peritonæum. And yet the majority of the teaching
in our medical colleges tends to disparage Hypogastric Lithotomy.[†] Why this
is so, I cannot understand, but the fact remains. The answer may be that
the rate of mortality is very much against the operation. This may be, for
reasons already given, but in Dulles's last table he makes the ratio *one in ten,*
and from the previous chapter we make it about equal to the lateral.
The fact is, as the operation stands before the profession, the rate of mortality
ought to be far greater than by other methods, for the simple reason that the

---

[*] Lithotomy and Lithotrity Compared, etc., by Thomas King, M.D., M.R.C.S., Surgeon to his Excellency
the French ambassador, etc., London, 1832, p. 330; Medico-Chirurgical Review, 1832, p. 42.

[†] As an exception, we refer the reader to the last edition of Bryant's Practice of Surgery, wherein the
American editor distinctly states that he always instructs his classes in the method of performing the hypogastric section.

very worst cases are those which have often been assigned to it. When perineal section has failed, or when lithotrity has been unavailing, then as a last
resort the hypogastric method is brought into requisition. This indeed is the
teaching of the colleges and the textbooks, and the figures allowed to stand in
the tables as *fair* representatives of the value of the operation. A short time
since Dr. Keyes (perhaps in answer to a reviewer of Dr. L. A. Stimson's work
on *Operative Surgery*, who asks, "How often Dr. Keyes has made suprapubic
lithotomy?"),* in a report to the New York Pathological Society,† detailed
three cases of death following the suprapubic operation, stating that up to that
period he had operated by lithotomy and lithotrity thirty-eight times and lost
four cases; three being the result of the suprapubic method. The latter cases I
give somewhat in detail, and as a sample of the kind that are generally referred
to the hypogastric section. In the first case, the patient was seventy-five years
old. In 1877, stone caught and measured 1¼ to 1¾ inches. "*The nervous, irritable temperament of the patient and the size of the stone* rendered lithotrity undesirable, and lithotomy was proposed but declined by the patient."‡ Two
months and a half later, the patient's symptoms became more distressing, "and
the suprapubic operation was performed." . . . . . "The whole operation
occupied less than half an hour." The patient died on the third day. In
the second case, a man, aged seventy-three, had been cut sixteen years previously in the perinæum and six phosphatic calculi removed. "He had
atony of the bladder." . . . "The urine contained albumen and casts, and there
was much cystitis." He was sounded and the instrument "gently introduced,"
and yet the patient "was *laid up for two weeks*, as the result of this *explora-
tion, and no operation was advised*." His sufferings, however, continued to tor-
ment him until he demanded relief. A lithotrite was therefore passed, one
stone was caught, crushed once, and nothing more attempted. This operation aggravated the cystitis, and *then* the suprapubic operation was performed. The patient died on the seventh day, the autopsy showing granular
kidney and pyelitis. In the third case, the patient was sixty-five years old,
had been operated upon two years before in Bellevue Hospital by lithotrity, and
a stone of one and a half inches in diameter, composed of urates and uric acid,
caught and crushed several times. The size and hard sharp edges of the fragments caused some cystitis, and after a rest of a couple of weeks, Dr. Keyes
decided to give ether, and crush as much as possible at a single sitting, using
a new lithotrite of Reliquet's. "After a few fragments had been crushed, it
became evident that the blades were clogged. No efforts succeeded in getting rid
of the fragments, which filled the female blade. The instrument was therefore

---

* American Journal of the Medical Sciences, January, 1879, p. 210.
† New York Medical Record, January 25th, 1879, p. 234.
‡ The italics are the author's.

withdrawn, and *enough force had to be used during its extraction to divulse* (slightly) *the urethra* at its point of natural constriction, about two inches from the meatus. The *patient had a chill and did badly.*" *This cystitis increased* and suprapubic lithotomy was performed, drainage being managed by a convolvulus catheter passed through the bas-fond and out at the anus. The patient did not rally; death occurred on the second day, *and surgical kidney was found on both sides at the autopsy.* I leave any unprejudiced mind to decide whether such cases as these ought to be admitted into the tables, and whether they offer a fair estimate of the value of the operation.

In the first case, the patient was an old man (seventy-five years), with such an irritable temperament and such a large stone that lithotrity was undesirable, and lithotomy denied. Two months and a half afterwards, when his condition had become much worse, the suprapubic method was resorted to.

In the second case, the patient was nearly as old, had atony of the bladder, aggravated cystitis, albumen and granular casts in the urine, a urethra and bladder so sensitive that the *gentle introduction* of a lithotrite laid him up two weeks. Litholapaxy was afterward attempted and failed, and then hypogastric lithotomy performed. Of course he died; so he would after any other operation.

In the third case, the man was aged sixty-five; litholapaxy was attempted and failed; the urethra was divulsed in withdrawing the instrument; severe cystitis set in and he "did badly;" and then again the high operation was resorted to. I say again, of course the patient died.

The question is, ought the records of cases of this character dissuade the surgeon from attempting the operation in favorable cases? Advocates for epicystotomy have stated especially the character of cases that ought to be subjected to it, and I am quite sure, as I have already written in the preface, that there are a large number of cases of calculus in the bladder which should only be treated by crushing; when, however, the stone is large and hard, as in Dr. Doughty's case; when the patient is too young to allow large-sized instruments to pass the urethra, especially in those cases where there is such a sensitive canal that the mere *introduction* of a sound, or of the searcher, may be followed by a chill, urethral fever and death; where the stone, as in my fourth case, was sacculated behind the prostate; where there has been intense and prolonged cystitis, and in many cases of stone in females, hypogastric lithotomy is the operation which, in my judgment, ought to be attempted.

At the present writing, I am quite aware that the voice of the majority is rather against me, and when I come to examine into the reasons for this antagonism I really cannot find them tenable. The objections are mainly two, viz., peritonitis and urinary infiltration. Of course, at this era we leave out the accidents of bursting the bladder with injections, or tearing the peritonæum accidentally from the struggling of the patient; although, in reality, these are by no means fatal.

To show the opinion of those of the profession who have considered the subject with regard to the dangers of the operation, a few ancient and modern authorities are here inserted. Thus, Heister says, after alluding to the rather accidental and compulsory operation of Franco, that surgeons have been for the most part dissuaded from performing the suprapubic operation, "because a wound made in the superior or *membranous* portion of the bladder seemed to the ancients, since the time of Hippocrates, certainly fatal."[*]

Samuel Sharp,[†] who was a pupil of Cheselden, to whom this method of operation owes so much, condemns it for many reasons, but especially in cases "of indurated bladder, in which there is always more or less difficulty and danger; but it would be *frightful* in this, not only by reason of the necessity of wounding the peritonæum, but of the difficulty of coming at the stone." Holmes also says:[‡] "The main danger is that of wounding the peritonæum;" and, again, Spence speaks of the great risk of such an occurrence and of the intestines escaping.[§]

Pirrie[||] says, one of the immediate dangers of the operation is wounding the peritonæum, and one of the greatest objections is the danger of infiltration of urine into the cellular tissue around the anus. Gross writes,[¶] "The procedure is liable to be followed by the injury of the peritonæum and urinary infiltration." Bryant agrees with the above: "The causes of death appear to have been peritonitis and urinary infiltration."[**]

Hamilton uses the following expressive words: "There are two principal sources of danger in the high operation, namely, urinary infiltration and opening into the cavity of the peritonæum. The precautionary measures which are to be adopted to prevent the first will presently be described; with reference to the second, it must be admitted that it is in certain cases with difficulty avoided. We have seen it happen in the hands of an experienced and skilful surgeon, and that, too, when he had just assured us that there was no danger of this accident when proper care was employed."[††] Latta,[‡‡] thus writes: "In

---

* Id ipsum quidem magis ideo, quia vulnus in superiori, sive membranacea vesicæ parte factum veteribus, a tempore jam Hippocrates lithiferum utique videbater. Heister De Lithotomia, quia Lit. Alto ut Vocant, etc., Book I, p. 296.

† A Treatise on the Operations of Surgery. By Samuel Sharp, Surgeon to Guy's Hospital, London, 1747, p. 92.

‡ A Treatise on Surgery. Philadelphia, 1876, p. 816.

§ Lectures on Surgery. By James Spence, F.R.C.S.E. Edinburgh, 1871, vol. ii, p. 1241.

|| Principles and Practice of Surgery. By William Pirrie. London, 1873, p. 776.

¶ A System of Surgery. By Samuel D. Gross, M.D. Vol ii, p. 894.

** The Practice of Surgery. London, 1872, p. 559.

†† The Principles and Practice of Surgery. New York, 1872, p. 857.

‡‡ A Practical System of Surgery. By James Latta, Surgeon in Edinburgh. In three volumes. Edinburgh and London, 1795, vol. i, p. 432.

the high operation, it has been remarked that the wound, both in the bladder and in the external integument, is much more difficult to be healed than in any other way of operating."

Erichsen[*] also adds his testimony in the following words: "After the operation there will always be the risk of urinary infiltration into the cellular tissue, around the margins of the wound. Another cause of danger is the wounding of the peritonæum."

On the other hand, a few surgeons, as Parker, Günther, Nœggerath, Souberbeille, and especially Dulles, Rachel, Podoska, Trendelenberg, and Petersen, have upheld the performance of epicystotomy. Dr. Nœggerath says,[†] after detailing his method of operation: "We conclude, therefore, that the high operation for stone, in a general point of view, may be executed just as easily and safely as the lateral or perineal section, while it presents some striking advantages over these methods in performing it upon women and children," etc.

Parker considers the method the very best for removing stones from the female bladder.

Petersen thus formulates the conditions which are favorable: 1st. For large hard stones. 2d. Encapsuled stones, or stones lodged in saccules behind the prostate. 3d. Hypertrophied prostate. 4th. "Hæmorrhoids." 5th. "Very fat people." 6th. "Tumors of the bladder." 7th. "Impermeable stricture where it is desirable to pass a fine catheter."[‡]

Dr. Rachel writes: "Suprapubic lithotomy is no *dernier ressort*; it is a first-class operation, and ought to be recognized as such."[§]

Malgaigne,[||] in his celebrated thesis, presented to the Academy of Medicine at Paris, 1850, and which gained for him the Chair of Operative Surgery, in drawing a comparison between the different operations for the removal of stone, expresses the opinion, in which I heartily concur, that the high operation is by far the easiest, and is especially adapted for the removal of large stones, *even after lateral lithotomy has failed*. And that the ease and rapidity with which calculi are discovered and removed, the freedom from hæmorrhage, the little danger of making false passages, or laceration of the soft parts, all should render the operation worthy of the highest consideration. In the last American edition of Bryant's *Surgery*, the editor, after referring to the statistics of the operation as given by Dr. Dulles in his last table, says: "I am convinced the operation is a good one and should be frequently performed. I always teach it to my students in operative surgery."[¶] It is useless, however, to multiply

---

[*] The Science and Art of Surgery. Philadelphia, p. 928.

[†] Epicystotomy, with Report of a Successful Case. By E. Nœggerath. New York Medical Journal. January, 1858.

[‡] American Journal of the Medical Sciences, April, 1881, p. 573.

[§] American Journal of the Medical Sciences, January, 1879, p. 153.

[||] British and Foreign Medico-Chirurgical Review, vol. vi, 1850, pp. 34, 38.

[¶] Bryant's Practice of Surgery, edited by John B. Roberts, A.M., M.D., Philadelphia, 1881.

quotations on this point; all surgeons appear to be agreed that the chief sources of danger are but two, these being peritoneal inflammation and urinary infiltration. To satisfy my mind on these points, and to ascertain the height to which the bladder will rise above the pubes at various ages, and how much of the apex of the viscus is generally covered with peritonæum, as well as to observe the character of the connective tissue behind the bones, I had the following experiments made on the cadaver. These dissections were made for me by Dr. McDowell, at the hospital on Ward's Island, the whole I think making a valuable table for the anatomist as well as for the surgeon who desires to attempt suprapubic lithotomy. I am, however, very well aware that these experiments are to be taken with a degree of caution, and must only be regarded as comparative, because in many cases of stone, in which the patients have suffered for a considerable time, the bladder is able to retain much less urine than during health. Yet it is interesting and instructive to the surgeon about to perform suprapubic lithotomy to know that in ordinary cases there will be sufficient space to allow him to remove a large stone without touching the peritonæum, even after most aggravated symptoms have continued for years. It may be well to note in this place, that Petersen, always an advocate for suprapubic lithotomy, proposes not only to distend the bladder but the rectum also, after the manner of Braune, and thus still further push up the serous coating of the intestines.

Experiment I.

Female, age 34; the bladder was injected until it reached 5 inches above the pubes, and was within 2 inches of the umbilicus. In this position the reflection of the peritonæum was 2½ inches above the superior border of the pubes, and the intervening space was filled by connective and cellular tissue only:

Experiment II.

Male, age 37; the bladder was injected (24 oz.) until distended; it reached 4 inches above the pubes and within 2 inches of the umbilicus. Here the duplication of the peritonæum from the anterior wall of the bladder on to the inner surface of the abdominal walls did not reach within 2½ inches of the upper border of the pubes.

Experiment III.

Male, age 50; 32 ounces water injected into bladder, it then reached 5 inches above the pubes, and within ½ inch of the umbilicus. In this position the duplication of the peritonæum was 2½ inches above the superior border of the pubes.

Experiment IV.

Male, age 26; injected 28 ounces of water into the bladder with moderate force. The bladder mounted 4 inches above the pubes. Transverse diameter

PLATE I.

Vide Experiment XI. page 58

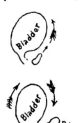

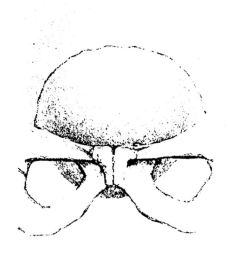

Experiment IV. page 56.

of the bladder, 4 inches. The lower margin of the peritonæum was 2½ inches above the pubes; it described a gentle curve, going below the internal abdominal ring on each side. Injected from 54 to 60 ounces of water with considerable force, when the bladder gave way between the pubes and the fold of peritonæum.

Experiment V.

Male, age 27; injected 30 ounces of water into the bladder. The bladder mounted 5 inches above the pubes, its transverse diameter being 3½ inches. Space between the pubes and peritonæum, 2½ inches.

Experiment VI.

Male, age 30; injected 25 ounces of water into the bladder. The summit of the bladder was 3½ inches above the pubes. Transverse diameter, 3½ inches. Distance between the pubes and peritonæum, 1½ inches. On the left of the median line the peritonæum made a rapid descent toward the pubes, while on the right it maintained its height for 1½ inches, and then descended abruptly. Injected from 60 to 63 ounces, when the bladder gave way at a point above the lower line of the peritonæum.

Experiment VII.

Male, age 30; injected 26 ounces of water into the bladder. Summit of the bladder rose 4 inches above the pubes. Transverse diameter of the bladder, 3½ inches. Peritonæum to pubes, 1½ inches. The lower margin of the peritonæum was irregular, being lower on the left side than the right, forming an angle a little to the left of the median line. There were no signs of previous inflammation.

Experiment VIII.

Male, age 39; injected 27 ounces of water into bladder. Bladder rose 4½ inches above pubes. Transverse diameter of bladder, 3½ inches. Space between the pubes and peritonæum, 2½ inches. Margin of peritonæum in a short curve, meeting the pelvis 1½ inches from the symphysis on either side. Injected from 55 to 60 ounces of water, when the walls of the bladder gave way at two points, side by side, on the superior surface.

Experiment IX.

Male, age 40; injected 22 ounces of water. Bladder rose 4 inches above pubes. Transverse diameter, 3½ inches. From pubes to peritonæum, 1½ inches. The fold of peritonæum was almost a straight line at right angles with the median line.

Experiment X.

Male, age 45; injected 19 ounces of water; bladder above pubes, 3 inches; transverse diameter, 3½ inches; pubes to peritonæum, 1½ inches; again injected 24 ounces; bladder above pubes, 3½ inches; transverse diameter, 3¾ inches; pubes to peritonæum, 1⅛ inches.

Experiment XI.

Male, age 47; injected 32 ounces of water into the bladder. Bladder mounted 3 inches above the pubes. Transverse diameter of bladder, 4½ inches. The bladder did not project anteriorly as in other cases. Usually when being injected, the anterior surface of the bladder rotates from below upwards, the portion of the bladder walls behind the pubes rising upwards, but in this case the portion behind the pubes remained stationary, so that the bladder appeared to rotate in the opposite direction. When injected, *the peritonæum did not rise at all from the pubes.* There were no adhesions of the bladder, peritonæum, or pubes; they separated on slight traction. No thickening or discoloration of parts, and no known history of inflammatory disease.

Experiment XII.

Male, age 49; injected into bladder, 26 ounces; bladder rose 4½ inches above the pubes; space between the pubes and fold of peritonæum, 2 inches.

Experiment XIII.

Male, age 50; injected water, 24 ounces; bladder above pubes, 4½ inches; transverse diameter, 4 inches; pubes to peritonæum, 2⅛ inches.

Experiment XIV.

Male, age 57; injected 22 ounces; bladder above pubes, 3½ inches; transverse diameter, 3¾ inches; pubes to peritonæum, ⅝ inch; again injected, 32 ounces; bladder above pubes, 4½ inches; pubes to peritonæum, 1¾ inches.

Experiment XV.

Male, age 65; injected 27 ounces of water. Bladder rose 3½ inches above the pubes; it was somewhat conical in shape, the apex projecting anteriorly and being 1¼ inches above the level of the pubes (body horizontal). Transverse diameter of bladder was 4½ inches. The lower margin of the peritonæum was irregular, being higher at one point than at another. (See diagram.) At the highest point it was 1¾ inches above the pubes, and at the lowest 1⅛ inches. Between the lower point and the pubes, the connective tissue was tense; it was not thickened, and gave way on slight traction; the peritonæum appeared

PLATE II.

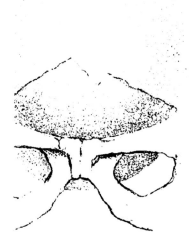

Experiment 15 page 58.

normal. Again injected 40 ounces water; the bladder rose 4¾ inches above the pubes; transverse diameter of bladder, 4¾ inches; lower margin of peritonæum nearly regular and 2¼ inches above the pubes; injected from 55 to 60 ounces, when the bladder gave way between the pubes and peritonæum.

Experiment XVI.

Male, age 72; injected 28 ounces of water into the bladder; bladder rose 4½ inches above pubes; space between pubes and peritonæum 2¼ inches.

Experiment XVII.

Female, age 30; injected 30 ounces water; bladder rose 3¾ inches above the pubes; space between pubes and the peritonæum, 1½ inches.

Experiment XVIII.

Female, age 30; injected 24 ounces of water; summit of the bladder was 4 inches above the pubes; transverse diameter 4½ inches; from pubes to peritonæum 3 inches. The uterus was enlarged, and there was some thickening of the peritonæum between the uterus and bladder. No evidences of cystitis or general peritonitis. Cause of death, carcinoma uteri.

Experiment XIX.

Female, age 34; injected 28 ounces; bladder above pubes, 3¾ inches; transverse diameter, 3¼ inches; pubes to peritonæum, 1½ inches; injected, 35 ounces; bladder above pubes, 4 inches; pubes to peritonæum, 1¾ inches. Lower margin of the peritonæum curved as usual.

Experiment XX.

Female, age 40; injected 28 ounces; bladder above pubes, 4½ inches; transverse diameter, 4 inches; pubes to peritonæum, 2 inches. The folds of the peritonæum extended across almost in a straight line.

Experiment XXI.

Female, age 43; injected 28 ounces; bladder above pubes, 4 inches; pubes to peritonæum, 1½ inches. Lower margin of peritonæum curved.

Experiment XXII.

Female, age 24; injected 20 ounces water; bladder mounted 3½ inches above the pubes; space between pubes and the peritonæum, 2¼ inches; again injected 40 ounces, when the peritonæum was 3¼ inches above the pubes.

Experiment XXIII.

Female, age 47; injected 26 ounces; bladder above pubes, 3¾ inches; transverse diameter, 4 inches; pubes to peritonæum, 1¾ inches. The lower margin of the peritonæum met the pelvic brim about two inches from the symphysis on the right side; on the left it described a shorter curve, coming one inch from the symphysis.

Experiment XXIV.

Female, age 50; injected 25 ounces; bladder above pubes, 4¼ inches; transverse diameter, 4 inches. *The peritonæum extended to the pubes.* It was very much thickened, of a yellow color, very dull in appearance; the bladder walls were not appreciably thickened. Water withdrawn, and bladder again injected; when 35 ounces had been injected, the adhesions between the peritonæum and pubes were torn apart by hand, it requiring considerable force to do so. After this, continuing to inject, the peritonæum rose from the pubes as in other subjects. When from 60 to 65 ounces had been injected, the bladder ruptured a little below the middle of the anterior surface.

Experiment XXV.

Female, age 76; injected 27 ounces; bladder above pubes, 3¾ inches; transverse diameter, 4¼ inches; pubes to peritonæum, 2 inches; again injected 35 ounces; bladder above pubes, 4¾ inches; transverse diameter, 5 inches; pubes to peritonæum, 2¾ inches.

Quantity of Water Injected till Bladder Ruptured.

	Number of ounces.
Case 4,	54 to 60
" 6,	60 to 63
" 8,	55 to 60
" 15,	55 to 60
" 24,	60 to 65
Average,	59¼ ounces.

Quantity of Urine Retained in the Bladder till there was Urgent Desire to Urinate.

Case 1, age 19,	16 ounces.
" 2, " 25,	12 "
" 3, " 26,	10 "
" 4, " 28,	13 "
" 5, " 39,	8 "
" 6, " 40,	10 "
" 7, " 45,	8 "
" 8, " 56,	8 "

By carefully reading over the table annexed, it will be seen that opportunity thus far has not allowed the dissection of any subjects younger than twenty-six years of age, but I am in hopes ere long to present some further experiments in this direction. However, in this patient, tabulated as Case 4, the bladder rose above the pubes 4 inches, 2⅜ inches being uncovered by peritonæum. In the oldest patient (case 25, aged seventy-six years), the bladder rose 4½ inches above the pubes, there being but two inches uncovered by the serous sac. In the former twenty-eight ounces of fluid were employed, in the latter twenty-seven.

Sex.	Age.	No. fl. oz. injected.	Height of bladder.	Transverse diameter.	Pubes to peritonæum.
Case 1, Male,	34	...	5	...	2½
" 2, "	50	32	5	...	2½
" 3, "	37	24	4	4	2½
" 4, "	26	28	4	4	2⅜
" 5, "	27	30	5	3⅝	2½
" 6, "	30	25	3½	3¼	1¾
" 7, "	30	26	4	3¼	1¾
" 8, "	39	27	4⅛	3¼	2¼
" 9, "	40	22	4	3½	1¼
" 10, "	45	24	3½	3¾	1⅛
" 11, "	47	32	3	4½	0
" 12, "	49	26	4½	...	2
" 13, "	50	24	4¼	4	2⅛
" 14, "	57	32	4¼	4¼	1¾
" 15, "	65	27	3½	4½	1⅜
" 16, "	72	28	4¼	...	2¼
" 17, Female,	30	30	3¼	...	1½
" 18,* "	30	24	4	4½	3
" 19, "	34	28	3¾	3½	1½
" 20, "	40	28	4½	4	2
" 21, "	43	28	4	...	1½
" 22, "	45	20	3½	...	2¼
" 23, "	47	26	3¾	4	1¾
" 24,* "	50	25	4⅛	4	0
" 25, "	76	27	3¾	4½	2
Average, . .	$43\frac{14}{25}$	$26\frac{12}{24}$	$4\frac{1}{25}$	$3\frac{43}{144}$	$2\frac{3}{92}$

In case No. 2 (a man aged forty-seven years), the anatomical conformation was very remarkable. The bladder rotated from behind forward, so that the anterior wall was completely covered by peritoneal investment, the contrary of which is found in the majority of cases, and this occurred, as Dr. McDowell remarks, without thickening or discoloration of parts or of any known history of inflammatory disease.

In case No. 24 (a woman aged fifty years), there was also no portion of the bladder which became uncovered with the membrane; on the contrary it extended to the pubes. By referring to this case, it will be seen that all the appearances of old pelveo-peritonitis were apparent.

* Peritonitis.

In case No. 17 (a woman aged thirty), with the injection of thirty ounces of fluid, the bladder rose three and three-quarters inches above the pubes, but left one and a half inches between the pubic symphysis and the duplicature of the peritonæum.

In the fifteen male cases recorded, there were six in which the bladder when injected did not rise uncovered to two inches, eight in which the space between the pubes and the anterior fold of the peritonæum was between two and three inches, and one in which the bladder was entirely covered anteriorly by the membrane.

Leaving out, then, the latter, as an anatomical anomaly the average space which is free from the peritonæum above the pubes in the injected bladder is within a small fraction of two inches.

It will also be remarked that there will be a space of about four inches of bladder-wall above the pubes, if the size of the stone necessitates an extension of the incision above the line of peritoneal reflection.

ADVANTAGES.

The advantages claimed for the suprapubic method are, first, the absence of danger from hæmorrhage. From this, however, it must not be inferred that there is no bleeding whatsoever, because very frequently there is quite a profuse discharge of blood from the incised bladder-wall, especially if the mucous membrane is sensitive and congested. A needle-puncture sometimes gives rise to a considerable flow of blood, as I have observed in some cases of vesico-vaginal fistula,* and therefore, if it be possible, when the incision into the bladder is being brought together, the needle should be carried through the thickness of the bladder, but brought out at the verge of the mucous lining. These bleedings, however, cannot be of much moment, for there are no vessels of any magnitude divided either in the incision in the linea alba, or the division of the bladder-wall, unless there be an anomalous course of the arteries and veins, and I am disposed to think this must have been the condition where such hæmorrhage has occurred, these cases being very few.

The next great advantage in the performance of hypogastric lithotomy is that of being able to *see* the different steps of the operation. No matter to what degree of perfection the *tactus eruditus* may have been cultivated, it is much more satisfactory to have "your eye upon" all the manipulations of knife and forceps. In the lateral operation, after the bulb of the bistoury or gorget has entered the groove in the staff, which indeed must be found by feeling, the operator can actually *see* nothing more of the procedure. The blade enters the bladder unseen, the finger enlarges the opening through the

---

* M. Cazenave was compelled to perform the hypogastric section to remove clots of blood which had formed from a simple puncture. Bulletin Méd. de Bordeaux, 1833. p. 82. Quoted by Velpeau.

prostate, the forceps are passed in and withdrawn with "touch" alone to guide them, while in the hypogastric section every step of the performance is assisted by the sense of sight, and an immense assistance it is. Another point of superiority in epicystotomy, is that it admits of the removal of stones of greater magnitude than by any other method, as is conclusively proven by many cases in which it has been successfully performed when the perineal methods and litholapaxy have failed..

Again, the accidents of wounding the rectum, of incontinence of urine, of impotence, of urinary fistulæ, are not to be feared as resulting from the method of Franco, while some or all of them may follow the other and more popular methods of removing calculi from the bladder through the perinæum. The main objections, as have already been fully considered in the first portion of this chapter, are urinary infiltration and peritonitis, which latter, as statistics prove, is rather rare, and it appears to me, need scarcely happen, unless there is an abnormal direction given to the peritonæum as the bladder rises above the pubes, as in one of the experiments made upon the cadaver.

CHAPTER IV.

CASES OF SUPRAPUBIC LITHOTOMY.

UNTIL about two years ago, whenever a case manifesting the symptoms of vesical calculus, of sufficient definiteness to suggest the thought of lithotomy, was presented to my notice, the idea of the operation was at once associated with one or other of the methods performed through the perinæum. In fact, having been taught, and read almost universally, that suprapubic lithotomy was obsolete and only to be undertaken under most peculiar circumstances, and having accepted the tradition without inquiry and without much thought, lithotomy, to my mind, meant perineal section, either lateral, bilateral, or median, for the removal of stone in the bladder. The proper estimation of the suprapubic method forced itself upon my mind, from the perusal of cases in which, from enlargement of the prostate or the magnitude of the calculus, the perineal operation, which had been actually commenced, had to be abandoned for the suprapubic, which was performed with success; and because in most of the modern works upon surgery, the high operation is only recommended for such extreme cases.

Thus in a case of impacted calculus weighing eight and one-half ounces, it was impossible to remove the stone through the perinæum, and the high operation was resorted to with success.* Samuel Cooper also thus writes: "Deschamps mentions an instance, in which M. Lassus, after using Hawkins's gorget, could not draw out the calculus, and he therefore immediately did the high operation, and the patient recovered."† Still more interesting is the fact that Franco, the author of the operation, was first led to perform it, for similar reasons, in the year 1560, as reported by Heister, as already noted in the chapter upon the history of this operation. Velpeau‡ disbelieves the latter statement, although he gives us no authority for his assertion. Liston§ also records a similar case, as does also Eve,‖ and the case of Krimer, in which a stone of twenty-three ounces was removed by the suprapubic method, after the failure of the perineal section the day before, is well known.¶

I have also witnessed lately a similar case in the hands of Dr. Doughty, in which Bigelow's litholapaxy failed, and an enormous stone was removed by the

---

* *Vide* Dulles, Suprapubic Lithotomy, American Journal of the Medical Sciences, April, 1878, p. 401.
† Cooper's Surgical Dictionary, Article Lithotomy.   ‡ Operative Surgery, vol. iii, p. 952.
§ Practical Surgery, p. 409.   ‖ Remarkable Cases in Surgery, p. 624.
¶ American Journal of the Medical Sciences (Dulles), 1875, p. 41.

high operation with success.* Erichsen also refers to two cases, and one has occurred to myself. *Vide* Case IV, page 73.

The inferences from such cases as these might certainly be that if suprapubic lithotomy were successful in such extremities, why would it not be appropriate in those cases where no such obstacles existed? And if the statistics of these operations, as presented in most of the modern surgical works, are drawn from such records, do they represent fairly the value of the method?

Shortly after this, the following cases came under my observation:

CASE I.—I. I. S., aged fifty-three years, *weight two hundred and forty pounds*, florid complexion, and nervous temperament, consulted Dr. Henry Minton, of Brooklyn, for a trouble of the urinary bladder of several years' duration. Some years since, the patient had suffered from internal hæmorrhoids, with occasional hæmorrhages from the rectum, complicated with a fistula in ano, which was operated upon with the knife and healed rapidly. Five years after, a second fistula appeared, which was cured by the internal administration of medicine. When I visited the patient, I found him in apparently good health, with a moderate appetite, and no inconvenience, save the frequent and persistent desire to urinate, which, gradually increasing for the past three years, had become almost unbearable. From time to time the urine passed had contained blood, for which he had also received treatment. He presented all the ordinary symptoms of stone, such as aching pain in the small of the back, drawing in the groin, pains in the perinæum, and uneasiness at the end of penis. When urinating, he would relieve the vesical tenesmus, which was very great, by bending the body forward and pressing his fingers upon the perinæum with great force. He had a pricking sensation at the neck of the bladder and elongation of the prepuce. In fact his physician had diagnosed the presence of a calculus, and called the consultation in regard to the propriety of its removal. Upon introducing the sound, there was such severe vesical spasm, that although the offending substance was detected, it was thought best, as my time was then limited, to make a more thorough examination, with the patient fully etherized, on the day but one following. A portion of his urine however, gave the following analysis: Sp. gr. 1018; reaction, acid; no sugar; a trace of albumen; sediment bulky and heavy, with a large amount of isolated and aggregated pus-corpuscles; one crystal of the triple phosphates.

This, as will be seen, was rather negative in its results, so far as the presence of the calculus was concerned. At the appointed time, the patient was thoroughly anæsthetized, the bladder was injected with a few ounces of water, at body temperature, and a calculus, an inch and three quarters in length, was found, resting on the left side of the bottom of the bladder. After due con-

---

* The reader is referred to Case V in this chapter.

sultation, I concluded to perform lateral lithotomy, not only because my experience was larger with that method than with any other, but because I had not lost a patient therefrom. The time was then appointed for the operation, but in the interval I again referred to the literature of epicystotomy, and after a good deal of thought, and I must own with some misgivings, determined to alter my mind, and to extract the stone above the pubes. The operation certainly appeared theoretically the simplest and the least dangerous, the objections to it, as laid down by all writers, being more apparent than real. In these days of ovariotomy, laparotomy, and excision of the rectum, a wound of the peritonæum is by no means fatal, and urinary infiltration, although an untoward accident, may be prevented, and is quite as likely to happen after the perineal section. Still, the very facts, that the opinions of the majority of the profession were opposed to the suprapubic method; that I had performed lateral and median lithotomy successfully; and above all, in case of an unfavorable result, the censure which would probably be cast upon the operator, not only by the friends and relatives of the patient, but by his own conscience for having departed from the beaten track and sacrificed a life to his temerity, were sufficient to cause considerable anxiety regarding the termination of the case.

However, fortified by late statistics,* on the 13th of May, 1878, at 3.15 o'clock P.M., assisted by Drs. Burdick, Richardson and Minton, and in the presence of several medical students, the operation was performed as follows: All the instruments, bed-clothing, vessels and sponges being "listered," and the atmosphere of the room charged with thymol spray, 1 to 100, the patient was placed on the table on his back, and ether administered. When the anæsthesia was complete, he was as usual, sounded, all the gentlemen present hearing the click and feeling the stone. The sound, No. 14 English scale, was then withdrawn, and a catheter of the same calibre, to the end of which a stopcock was attached, was introduced into the bladder, which was then thoroughly washed out and injected with carbolized water, 1 to 100, at a temperature of 98½°. The bladder was filled by means of a good-sized syringe, holding about four ounces, and about twelve ounces were injected into the viscus.

The stopcock was then turned, the catheter was held at a right angle with the pubis, and retained in this position by an assistant encircling the penis with the forefinger and thumb to prevent the escape of fluid by the side of the catheter.

An incision was then made, about four inches in length, in the linea alba, to the root of the penis. It was necessary to enlarge this integumental cut during the operation, on account of the immense amount of adipose tissue beneath the skin. As soon as the abdominal cavity was opened, a mass of fat presented at the wound, which, as in Dr. Rachel's case, prolonged the operation somewhat;

---

* The tables of Suprapubic Lithotomy show a mortality of but 1. in 9.7. *Vide* page 47.

the delay being occasioned by the anxiety to avoid the peritonæum or the omentum, to which these masses of fat might have been attached. Cutting carefully through this layer brought the bladder to view. The handle of the catheter was then depressed between the legs of the patient, and its point made to press upon the anterior wall of the bladder. The point of the finger was then inserted into the wound, which was at least three inches in depth, and by moving the catheter the correct relation of the parts was distinctly made out. The lips of the wound were then carefully held aside with retractors, and a good-sized curved needle, threaded with a double carbolized catgut ligature, was passed through the upper portion of the bladder, drawn through and tied in a loop; the needle was cut off, and the loop hooked upon the finger of a trusty assistant. At this stage of the operation, the patient, very plethoric, became almost asphyxiated; the face was perfectly purple, respiration ceased, and the pulse was feeble and intermittent. Within five minutes, by drawing the tongue forward with a tenaculum, and performing artificial respiration (Sylvester's method), the symptoms subsided, and the operation was continued. By turning the stopcock fixed at the end of the catheter, about one-third the quantity of water was allowed to escape from the bladder in order to prevent too much of a gush of fluid when the viscus was incised; and, to render the recti tense, the legs of the patient were allowed to fall over the edge of the table, thus bringing the muscular walls of the abdomen down upon the bladder, with a view of also preventing the water from flowing into the abdominal cavity. Although, from experience in ovariotomy, such an occurrence would not have probably occasioned inconvenience, still these precautions at that time were deemed necessary.

A curved bistoury was then introduced in front of the loop of catgut, and the bladder incised toward the pubes. A small quantity of the carbolized water gushed out, and being caught with sponges did not pass into the abdomen. I did not, as has been recommended, follow the course of the bistoury with my finger, nor was the stone whirled up to the opening made in the bladder. When the parts were all dry, I inserted my finger into the bladder, distinctly felt the stone lying on the right side of the prostate, and with a pair of lithotomy forceps extracted it without any difficulty. The catheter was withdrawn from the bladder as soon as the incision had been made in the viscus. The loop of catgut was then drawn well up, to bring the lips of the bladder wound well into view, which was closed with fine carbolized catgut sutures, the ends of the threads being cut off close to the knots. The loop of catgut was then slackened, and the bladder allowed to drop into position; sufficient traction, however, being made to prevent a complete approximation of the vesical walls. The loop was then secured at the upper angle of the wound, and the abdominal incision closed with silver-wire sutures passing through the entire abdominal walls, integument, fat, and muscular tissue. An inch, however, at the lower end of the cut was allowed to remain open for drainage, and a good-sized carbolized tent inserted into the opening. As the anæsthesia was passing off symptoms of vesical tenesmus of a violent character presented, for which, at 4.45 P.M., tinc. hyos., gtt. xv, were given.

At 5 P.M., and after the patient had been placed in bed, the pulse was 68, and the temperature was 97°. At 5.15, the vesical tenesmus appeared to threaten again, when the dose of hyoscyamus was repeated. Shortly after the second dose this symptom entirely disappeared.

At 8 o'clock P.M., there was a sudden desire to urinate, and a small quantity of urine was passed through the urethra. In an hour the catheter was introduced and six ounces of urine drawn.

At midnight two ounces of water were drawn with the catheter; the pulse was 84, and the temperature $99\frac{3}{5}$°. Had slept quietly for two hours.

May 14th, second day, 5 o'clock A.M.: Temperature $99\frac{1}{2}$°; pulse 92; water drawn.

At 7 o'clock A.M., night-dress and bedclothes changed without trouble. The patient was bright and cheerful, having nothing of which to complain.

During the night there was occasionally a discharge of urine from the wound.

At 5 o'clock P.M.: Temperature $100\frac{4}{5}$°; pulse 95. Urine drawn every two hours.

May 15th, third day, 10 o'clock A.M.: Temperature $99\frac{4}{5}$°; pulse 88.

At 5 o'clock P.M.: Pulse 104, temperature $100\frac{4}{5}$°. Discharge from wound somewhat offensive.

On the morning of the 16th I received the following word from Dr. C. W. Cornell, who had the patient entirely in charge during my absence: "Mr. S. passed a better night than last, sleeping most of the time. Was not nearly so restless. Feels very comfortable this morning. The odor from the lower angle of the wound is still offensive. The discharge is, however, less. I removed the dressing this morning under the spray (thymol), not, however, removing the straps, but cleansing the parts between them. I change the seton quite often, thoroughly cleansing the parts at the same time. Urine has been drawn regularly, and is about the same in every respect."

On the 17th, fifth day, I cut out the catgut suture holding up the bladder. On the 18th, sixth day, the report was: "The patient slept very well. The discharge is about the same in quantity and character. The urine still escapes from the wound, causing considerable discomfort. The probe can be passed down between the lips of the wound about $3\frac{1}{2}$ inches. This morning, according to directions, I coated the line of incision with collodion, and should judge from appearances that the wound has united along its entire upper portion.

PLATE III

Case I. J.S. Travelling agent, age 53 years,
Weight 240 ℔. (page 69)

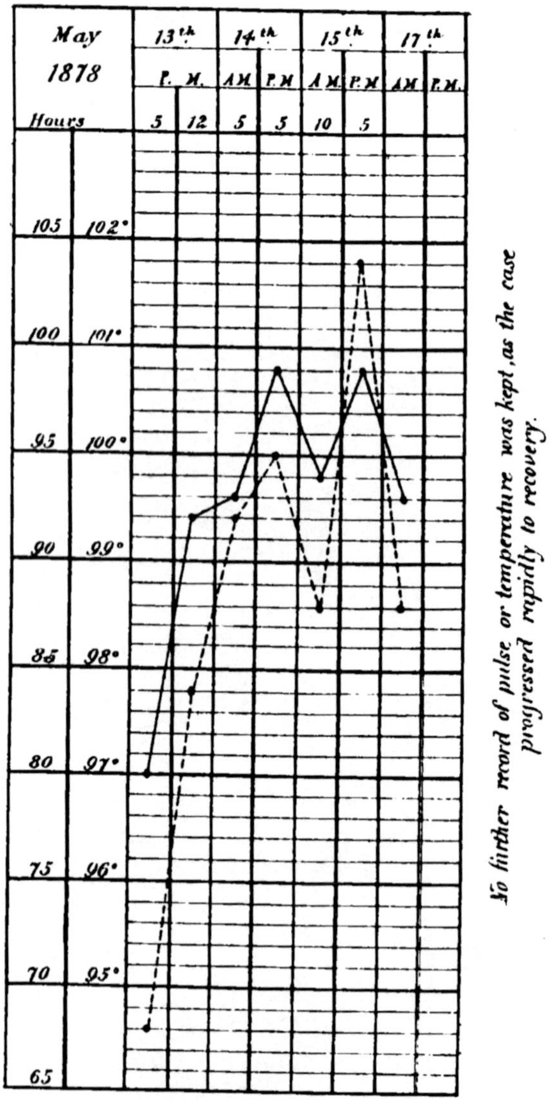

May 1878		13th		14th		15th		17th	
		P. M.		A.M.	P.M.	A.M.	P.M.	A.M.	P.M.
Hours		5	12	5	5	10	5		
105	102°								
100	101°								
95	100°								
90	99°								
85	98°								
80	97°								
75	96°								
70	95°								
65									

No further record of pulse or temperature was kept, as the case progressed rapidly to recovery.

The dotted line represents the pulse.

Temperature and pulse remain the same, the former being 99⅗°, the latter 88. No untoward symptoms have developed. Catheter is passed every three hours."

On the 19th, the seventh day, I removed the wires, and, as a matter of experiment, and to ascertain if I could reach the bladder above the pubes and thus _make drainage, I ordered a catheter placed in the wound instead of the tent, and to have it retained there by means of lint packed around it. On May 21st, I received the following from Dr. Cornell: " Patient passed a most comfortable night, and is in as good, if not better, condition than when you saw him. I have placed a catheter in the wound, and packed the lint around it. I first placed dry lint in the lower portion of the wound, and above this, lint saturated with oil, to prevent the absorption of urine. The packing was secured by strips of adhesive plaster. Since then there has been but a slight discharge. Very little, if any, of the urine, however, escaped through the catheter in the wound, most of it being drawn with the catheter. This morning I carefully examined the wound and find it thoroughly closed."

On the 12th day I removed all the packing and catheter, and allowed the patient to sit up. Occasionally—sometimes once a day, sometimes twice a day, sometimes once in three days—a little urine would escape from the wound ; but this soon passed away, and he was going about his room in four weeks, and soon attended to his regular business, and is to-day cured. The Plate will show the pulse and heat line of the patient. The calculus was a mixed one and weighed ℥iij ℈jss.

I have been, perhaps, somewhat too minute in the details of this case, but I have given it in full, because often the treatment was experimental, on account of the great diversity of opinions that exist regarding these very details ; some surgeons preferring that no sutures be used, the wound being allowed to take care of itself; others, that drainage should be made through the rectum, while others advise the permanent retention of the catheter.

This case must be regarded as rather a typical one, on account of the corpulence of the patient, which condition is said by some to contraindicate the operation.

CASE II.—Not very long after this time, and when I had made myself somewhat more familiar with the history of these operations, and had made an especial study regarding the duplications of the peritonæum over the bladder, a second case was sent to me, by Dr. John Butler, of this city (New York). This patient came from the country to Dr. Butler, to be treated for senile hypertrophy of the prostate. The doctor discovered, immediately upon introducing the catheter, the presence of a calculus, and asked me to take charge of the case. The patient was in his seventieth year, had always had good health, excepting of late, when he had trouble in passing his urine, with great urinary tenesmus, and sometimes complete retention. He had also suffered from stricture of the urethra, and had a false passage leading from the urethra to the right of the penis. He was of spare habit of body, but possessed apparently much vitality.

Although the age of this patient was rather against the success of the operation, yet his prostate was so enormously enlarged that I was well convinced I should have great trouble in completing any variety of perineal lithotomy, and therefore determined to resort to the high operation. According to the table of M. Belmas,* the proportion of deaths at this age, after suprapubic lithotomy, is 1 to 1⅔; and according to Rankin 1 in 3.80. *Vide* page 48.

On the 24th of December, at the Hahnemann Hospital, I performed the operation, assisted by Dr. John Butler and several medical students.

The same process as that I have already recorded was adopted. The bladder was injected with the carbolic water, 1 to 100, at a temperature of 98°, through the catheter fitted with a stopcock. I noticed upon attempting to distend the bladder, after 4 to 6 ounces of water were injected, that there appeared to be an obstacle to the further entrance of the fluid into the viscus, which I found afterwards was occasioned by the thickness of the walls of the bladder, and to the space occupied by the hypertrophied prostate.

The incision was commenced and carried in the same direction as before, and the usual amount of fat found upon the apex of the bladder. Upon incising the viscus, the stone, weighing about 190 grains, was readily extracted. Search was made for other calculi, but none were found. It was during this manipulation that I was able to ascertain the approximate size of the prostate, which appeared about that of a large orange, and felt like a fleshy tumor inside the bladder.

The vesical wound was carefully stitched with fine carbolized catgut ligatures, and the external cut brought together with silver-wire, excepting the lower angle, into which a tent saturated with carbolized vaseline was inserted.

At 5.30 o'clock P.M., the pulse was 68, temperature 98°.

At 7 o'clock P.M., pulse was 100, temperature 99½°.

At 12 o'clock, midnight, the pulse was 112, temperature 99½°.

On the 25th (Christmas day), at 9 o'clock A.M., pulse 122, temperature, 100°.

At 12 o'clock A.M., pulse 125, temperature 101¾°.

When I made my visit the pulse was weak; the patient had vomited. There was a thick coating upon his tongue, much thirst, a blueness around the eyes, a hectic flush upon his cheeks, and altogether the symptoms were not favorable. He was, however, rational, and answered questions well and promptly. His urine had been drawn regularly every two hours; none had escaped from the wound. I ordered the catheter (a soft Nélaton, with countersunk eye) to be retained in the bladder, and gave him, or rather ordered, aconite to be continued.

At 3 o'clock P.M., pulse 132, temperature 101½°.

* Traité de la Cystotomy Sus-pubienne. Paris, 1827, p. 91.

At 5.30 o'clock P.M., pulse 128, temperature 101°.

At 11 o'clock P.M., pulse 120, temperature $100\frac{2}{10}$°.

At 12 o'clock P.M., pulse 120, temperature $99\frac{1}{2}$°.

On December 26th, at 5 o'clock A.M., pulse 130, temperature 102°.

At 7 o'clock A.M., pulse 135, temperature $99\frac{8}{10}$°.

At 8 o'clock A.M., pulse 104, temperature $99\frac{8}{10}$°.

When I saw him this morning his appearance was about the same as when I had made my visit the night before. But his general aspect was not very favorable. ℞. Arsen. 3d, every hour.

The urine had escaped freely from the catheter. He had taken some milk, which he relished, but still had thirst and was very restless. Had, however, a good deal of sleep, but awakened unrefreshed. Wound was carefully dressed, all soiled linen, bandages and straps removed. Medicine continued.

At 4 o'clock, pulse and temperature about the same. Gave stimulants (brandy) frequently.

At 6 o'clock P.M., pulse 110, temperature 98°.

At 10 o'clock he appeared more quiet.

From 10.45 o'clock to 11.30 P.M. he slept. From 11.30 o'clock to 12.30 P.M. was awake; took some milk. The sheet being a little soiled was changed, the tent taken out and cleaned, and a powder of Arsen. 3d trit. given, which was to be repeated every hour, and stimulants *pro re nata*.

From 1 to 2 o'clock A.M., slept, took some milk and cracked ice with brandy. Vomited slightly. Pulse 104, temperature 97°. Catheter cleaned and a new carbolized tent introduced. No urine had escaped from the wound.

From 3 to 4 o'clock A.M. was restless, but slept a little. Pulse weak.

On 27th, 9 o'clock A.M., patient appeared to be sinking. His pulse was very weak, but not very rapid, beating at about 104, with a temperature of about 97°. There was some slight tympanitis, but no sensitiveness of the abdomen, in fact excepting the usual soreness attendant upon the wound, the sensitiveness of the parts had gradually diminished. Carbo veg. 6th was given every hour, and stimulants pushed as far as he could bear them. I may here state that from the first day he had been troubled with hiccough, which was temporarily arrested by Hyos. 3d in water. This symptom had now returned with renewed violence.

At 12 o'clock he appeared about the same with a slight fall in the temperature.

At 6 P.M., he was very restless and more sunken, with a pulse of 135, and a temperature of 96°. At 12 o'clock, pulse 140, temperature $96\frac{1}{2}$°. Very restless and some muttering, cold extremities and cold sweat upon the forehead.

On the 28th, at 12.05 o'clock, midnight, the pulse was 136, temperature 96°. No urine escaping from the catheter for the last two hours.

At 3.30 A.M., pulse 135, temperature 96°.

At 6 o'clock A.M., pulse 136, temperature 96°.

28th December, 7.30 A.M., pulse 124 and very faint, temperature 95°. Unconscious. (The Plate shows the lines of pulse and temperature.)

He died about 3 o'clock in the afternoon.

The post-mortem examination was made that evening, by myself, Drs. Butler and Dennison.

Rapid decomposition was taking place, and there was some air in the intestines. The incision in the abdominal walls had healed almost entirely, and there was a large amount of plastic material around and beneath the wound. The bladder wound had also closed for the most part. The lower portion of the incision, however, was open; in it a catgut ligature, somewhat softened, was found. The ligatures at the upper angle of the wound had almost entirely disappeared. The bladder was small, contracted, and very much thickened, and as before stated, the prostate, enormously enlarged, occupied the greater portion of the viscus. The peritonæum just above the wound was congested for the space of about half an inch, and then appeared perfectly healthy, as did all the other viscera examined.

Although this was an unfortunate ending to this case, it does not, to my mind, present any evidences against suprapubic lithotomy, and I felt the better satisfied that I had selected this method, after I had ascertained the size of the prostate. I scarcely think that I should have been able to extract the stone through such an enlarged and hardened mass. The patient died of exhaustion, as he would in all probability had the lateral or the median perineal section been performed. We must remember that at the age of this patient, the mortality by the ordinary methods is about 1 in 3⅓.*

CASE III.—U. P. W., was born in New York city, on March 10th, 1817, and lived his entire life in the vicinity. At the time of his demise, his age was sixty-two years, nine months, and six days. His health was always moderate, having been never confined to his bed up to one year prior to his death. His first indisposition occurred about 1858, he suffering at that time from dyspepsia, which continued for four or five years. In 1863, he was affected with hæmorrhoids, which troubled him for many years, and for which he underwent a great variety of treatment, with varied results, but without any permanent amelioration. In 1876, he was attacked with nephritic colic, and began passing uric acid calculi. In July, 1879, all the symptoms of stone manifested themselves in a most aggravated form, and for a relief of these symptoms he was sent to me. He was emaciated, passing putrid urine loaded with pus and blood-corpuscles, hyaline and granular casts, and epithelia from pelvis of kidney and ureter. The most aggravated suffering, however, was the

---

* Holmes's System of Surgery, vol. iv, p. 1061.

PLATE IV. page 72.

Case II. Patient aged 20 Years, farmer by occupation, suffered from stricture and false passages.

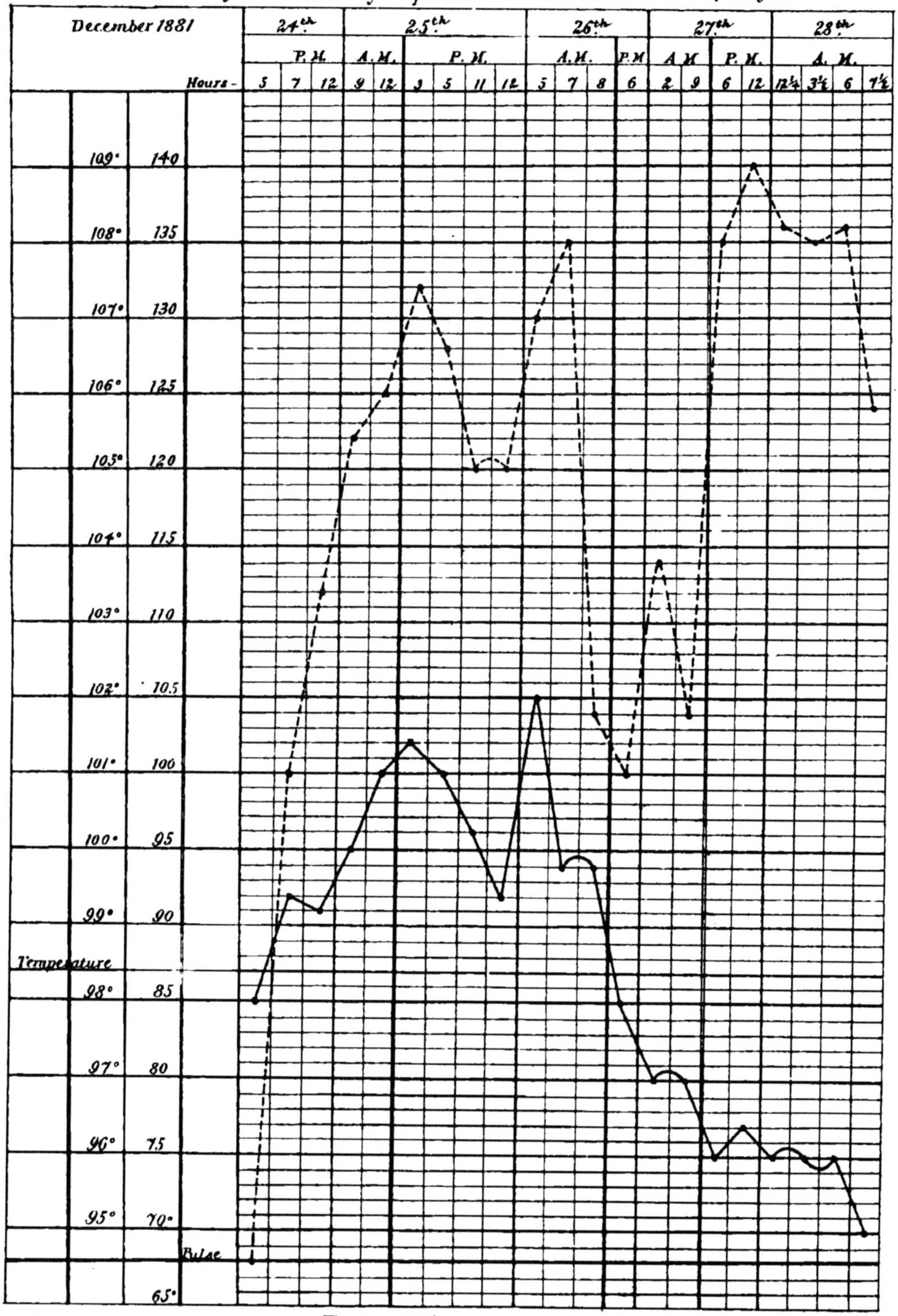
December 1881
24th
25th
26th
27th
28th
P. M.
A. M.
P. M.
A. M.
P. M
A. M
P. M.
A. M.
Hours -
5
7
12
9
12
3
5
11
12
5
7
8
6
2
9
6
12
12¼
3½
6
7½
109°
140
108°
135
107°
130
106°
125
105°
120
104°
115
103°
110
102°
105
101°
100
100°
95
99°
90
Temperature
98°
85
97°
80
96°
75
95°
70°
Pulse
65°

The dotted line represents the pulse.

terrible urinary tenesmus, strangury, and priapism, with bloody urine, which nothing but the largest doses of Morphia could relieve, and then he never was entirely free from suffering.

On December 13th, 1879, as a *dernier ressort*, he being in very bad condition for any operation whatsoever, and having a urethra so extremely sensitive that the passage of a soft flexible bougie would throw him into a chill, immediately followed by the most intense suffering, I concluded, at his request, to perform hypogastric lithotomy. The operation was readily accomplished after the manner laid down in the succeeding chapter, and three uric acid calculi extracted with the fingers, weighing ʒss, grains xij. But the condition of the mucous lining of the bladder was remarkable for its pulpy, dark-brown hue; the walls were immensely thickened, and the prostate much enlarged. The operation was completed at 3.30 P.M., having begun shortly after 2 o'clock, and there being several delays occasioned by the extreme prostration of the patient. From time to time, it was necessary to give him hypodermic injections of whiskey to restore the pulse, which on several occasions failed entirely.

At 5 P.M., his pulse was 98, temperature 95½°. Coldness over surface and somewhat wandering in mind. ℞. Aconite and Veratrum every two hours.

12, midnight, pulse 110, temperature 99°. Patient restless but more conscious, violent urinary tenesmus, and great pain in the wound. ℞. Hyos., gtt. xx, every three hours, in alternation with arsenic.

December 14th, 9 A.M., pulse 135, temperature 105.4°; almost unconscious; no urine from either catheter or wound. *Vide* Plate.

December 15th, died.

This was a rapid demise. The post-mortem appearances showed surgical kidney, trabeculated bladder, with immensely hypertrophied walls, which were covered on the outside with dark purple spots; the whole mucous membrane was pulpy and purple, and in a state of decomposition.

CASE IV.—The history of this case previous to the operation, is well described by the gentleman himself, who, in the following expressive letter, details the circumstances surrounding and the pain attending upon his case.

NEW YORK, January 3d, 1882.

DR. WILLIAM TOD HELMUTH.

DEAR SIR: Having suffered for several years, various pains connected with the bladder, scrotum, and glans penis, and being often compelled to micturate from ten to twelve times a day, the annoyance led me to consult with various laymen, as well as physicians, and also to refer to such medical works as would enlighten me upon the subject. Aconite, Rhus, Bryonia, Buchu, Ignatia, Mercurius, Colocynth, Phosphorus, Belladonna, Podophyllin, Lycopodium, Capsicum, and Nux vomica, were all taken, sometimes combined, and sometimes alternated. A physician of celebrity in this city stated that I had not a calculus, as my face did not indicate the presence of stone. I am nearly seventy years of age, never smoke or use tobacco or spirits, and have always lived a temperate life, my general health being excellent. About eighteen months since I was seized with a severe pain in my left side, followed by another attack about ten months after. In both these the suffering was most intense. In May, 1881, I visited New Haven, Connecticut (74 miles), and returned the same day. My business required that I should ride two or three hours about the city, and then having occasion to micturate, I observed that the urine was flecked with blood, which was the first evidence that there was anything seriously wrong with my bladder. A month or two later, after walking down Broadway to my store, about two miles from my house, I again passed blood from my bladder. From that period, my urine became a matter of study with me, and purchasing a dozen six-ounce large-mouthed white bottles, I micturated in them when at home, and allowed them to stand from one to two days or more, and watched the result. There was always some pain in the penis, and difficult micturition. I take at random from my note-book (March 8th, 1881), the periods at which I was obliged to urinate, passing from 1 to 3 or 4 ounces: "A.M., 3.30, 6, 8.10, 10.45; P.M., 12.50, 2.45, 4.50, 6.20, 7.45, 10, 11.05; thermometer 36°." There was always pain along the urethra and in the glans penis, and constant desire to urinate. I went with my family to Poland Springs, Maine, where the water is said to be pure and alkaline, and remained there two months. I found a large number of people afflicted with kidney or urinary troubles there, but of whose troubles one would know nothing unless drawn out in private conversation. Most of the visitors supposed they were benefited by the waters, and I found the rest and change favorable, but when body and mind were redirected to their accustomed employment, the recurrence of pain evinced the relief was temporary. At first, after much activity, the albumen in my urine was very marked, and taking it to my physician, he tested it with Nitric acid, and informed me that it was one-third albumen. It was examined by him several times, and when I was not actively employed, it was only slightly charged with mucus, but generally heavily loaded with albumen. Being anxious concerning my condition, I submitted my urine to a professional microscopist, who informed me that there were many casts found in it, and that I certainly was suffering from Bright's disease. Subsequently, however, the urine was examined by one of the most celebrated surgeons, who could not detect any casts, but found a large excess of uric acid. It was again examined in Boston, by a professed microscopist, who informed me there were no casts in my urine, but much uric acid. I suffered great agony from the jar of riding in a carriage, the urine being bloody, and I therefore concluded there was a calculus in my bladder; the idea had been suggested before, and I had been advised to be sounded. Having an aversion to this, supposing it to be more objectionable than it proved, and being worried by pain in the urethra and glans penis, and having to micturate frequently, at the solicitations of my friends, I called on Dr. T. F. Allen, who suggested immediate sounding, which being done, a calculus was found, which appeared to be encysted and not easy of access, and which my experience told me must be removed in time, or in time it would remove me.

Respectfully yours, etc.

Dr. Allen referred the patient to me; and, after carefully sounding him, I could detect with ease, a calculus, lying on the left of the prostate, which appeared immovable, and which from the peculiar nature of the " feel " given to the searcher indicated that a portion of it was covered by membrane.

At this period, as the urine was very ammoniacal, I therefore had the bladder washed out twice a day, with a saturated solution of the biborate of soda; and an analysis made which showed: color, amber; reaction, slightly acid; specific gravity, 1.020; albumen, ½ of 1 per cent.; pus-corpuscles very abundant; connective tissue in scanty shreds; epithelia, prostatic, vesical (middle and deep layers), pelvic, and renal.

The absence of acid constituents in this specimen was probably owing to the alkaline washings. On December 21st, 1881, I attempted litholapaxy, using Key's lithotrite. Do what I could, it was impossible to dislodge the calculus sufficiently to get it firmly within the jaws of the instrument; and though I could fasten the lithotrite upon the projecting portion of the stone, the blades would slip off, only taking off a small portion of the offending substance. In several instances I had firm hold of the stone, but from the "feel" imparted to my hand, I knew I had either the bladder-wall, or that portion of it covering the greater portion of the calculus within my grasp, and dared not risk turning the screw. The patient was turned on both sides, placed in the recumbent and semi-recumbent positions, but without avail; and, after an hour and a half's hard work, I was obliged, very much to my chagrin, to relinquish the operation.

Upon this, I determined to resort to the high operation, which was performed on the 18th of January, 1882. There was a large accumulation of fat over the bladder, and the superficial adipose tissue on the abdominal wall was very deep, the incision measuring in depth about five inches. Upon opening the bladder there was very profuse hæmorrhage, which being arrested, I introduced my fingers into the wound, and found the calculus lying deeply in the left side of the bas-fond, and almost completely encysted; after some difficulty I was enabled to turn it out with my fingers, and then easily withdrew it with the forceps. In this instance, instead of holding up the viscus with the curved needle, I employed forceps with catches at the handles, and with wide fenestrated blades. This method saved the puncture made in the wall of the vesica by the needle.

The calculus (composed of uric acid and ammonium urate), was horse-chestnut-shaped and was 5¼ inches in circumference, and 1 inch in diameter; weight, 620 grains. The bladder was closed with carbolized catgut, and the incision with silver wire. An india-rubber drainage-tube was introduced at the lower extremity of the wound, which was dressed with borated cotton and old linen, and washed with a weak solution of carbolic acid. The deeper portions of the cut were dressed with glycerine and carbolic acid. The incision was then properly strapped with adhesive plaster, the application of which was continued after sutures were taken out, and the straps covered with collodion, as was also the surface in the region of the incision; this was done to prevent excoriation from urine. The sutures were removed January 24th. The wound was dressed three times a day for the first week, and subsequently twice daily, except when copious discharges from the incision required additional attention. On January 31st, the drainage-tube was discontinued, and iodoform bougies, 5 grains each, were introduced regularly twice each day, in the entire depth of the cut. Patient sat up for the first time on January 30th, for about fifteen minutes, and on January 31st, for three hours (from 11 A.M.–2 P.M.), also from 4.30–7.30 P.M., making six hours in all.

February 12th, patient sat up for eleven hours, and walked at times during the day, thirty to forty-five minutes.

February 14th, remained out of bed for six hours, and walked for about half an hour about the room and in the hall.

The catheter was introduced at time of the operation (January 18th), and was removed and cleansed at each dressing for the first week, and subsequently every three hours.

On first sitting up in a chair (January 31st) the catheter was removed, but it was reintroduced again on lying down, and its use was steadily continued. On February 7th, india-rubber tubing was attached to the instrument, which acted as a siphon, and proved a great convenience. On February 8th, the use of the catheter was discontinued on account of the irritation of the urethra, the urine passing naturally.

Flow of Urine.—From January 18th to 21st, copious discharge of urine came from the wound, tinged with blood. On January 21st, the first clear urine passed from the catheter, making during the day (twenty-four hours) 1¼ pints. Other discharges as follows: January 23d, 1 pint, 15 ounces; January 24th, 2 pints; January 25th, 2 pints; January 26th, 2 pints; January 27th, 2 pints; January 28th, 1 pint, and much discharge from the incision; January 29th, 2 pints; January 30th, 2 pints; January 31st, 1 pint. Catheter out, and more discharged from the wound.

When less urine was passed, it was because a portion of it passed through the incision and could not be collected or measured. February 8th, catheter was removed, and 4 ounces of urine passed naturally by the urethra. February 10th, 23 ounces were voided naturally, the remainder coming through the cut. On February 12th, the water was passed naturally once in two hours, to prevent its escape through the wound.

Diet.—January 18th to 23d, barley-water every four hours, subsequently, with slight variations, as follows: 2 o'clock A.M., 7 ounces of barley-water; 6 o'clock A.M., 7 ounces of mutton and barley broth; 10 o'clock A.M., 2 lean mutton-chops, with Irish potatoes, Graham bread with butter, and black tea. A 2 o'clock P.M. (dinner), mutton, or fowl, and potatoes, baked apples, bread (always Graham), butter, and tea; 6 P.M., 7 ounces of mutton and barley broth, with some of the pieces of the mutton in it; 10 P.M., 7 ounces of mutton and barley broth, or barley alone if the mutton is too heavy. February 13th, exchanged the black tea for 7 ounces of milk.

State of Health.—First day, much nausea on recovering from effects of the ether. Second day, vomited 3½ pints of black bile. Third day, vomited 2¼ pints more. Fourth day, 1 pint more. Afterwards he was fed with and re-

tained barley-water till January 24th. No chill or indication of fever occurred. The sleep was first irregular, from four to eight hours, but as a rule the patient suffered no inconvenience from want of sleep.

February 11th, was awakened by nurse every two hours, that the urine might pass per urethram, and thus prevent any flow through the wound. After the operation the pain was acute for about twelve hours.

Action of Bowels.—First, on January 26th (eight days after operation), a full passage, using 12 ounces of tepid water. Second, four days later, using 10 ounces of water. Third, natural action, without any enema, and subsequently regular daily evacuations, using small enemata.

The patient steadily improved, and is now cured. I called upon him to-day, June 4th, and found him at his Sunday-school.

The following chart shows the pulse and temperature during his confinement within doors.

After this work had been completely prepared for the press, I opened the bladder (above the pubes) of a boy, aged five years, who I supposed was dying of rupture of the bladder, and who was almost pulseless when I placed him on the table. The case had been sent to my clinic, at the college, presenting all the symptoms of stone; the child rolling on the floor with agony when endeavoring to micturate, and then passing only small quantities of urine. He had also occasional hæmorrhage from his bladder, and was feverish and restless, with a pained expression of countenance. Withal he had an exceedingly elongated prepuce, the orifice being about the size of a needle. I sounded him at once, and could detect no calculus, but distinctly felt on the convex surface of the curve of the sound, just at the neck of the bladder, a rough and uneven surface,—just such a sensation as belongs to a trabeculated bladder from atony and long cystitis, and which I had often · recognized before. There was no sharp, metallic click, which immediately points to the presence of stone. I circumcised him at once, and for several days all his symptoms appeared to improve. In a fortnight he was brought back to the college in a most pitiable condition. I sent him to the hospital, and that afternoon (Saturday), in the presence of several medical gentlemen, easily detected the soft grating, or what I might call "mucoid sensation," with the sound. I then endeavored to draw off his urine with a fine flexible catheter, but only succeeded (he being under ether) in removing an ounce of water. On the next morning early, I was informed by the house surgeon that the boy had passed an agonizing night, that no water could be drawn from the bladder, and that he was rapidly sinking. I then endeavored to catheterize him, but found no urine. The bladder reached to the umbilicus and its anterior wall, hard, and apparently distended, could be felt beneath the integument. I introduced an aspirating needle at two points, but without effect, and as a last resort determined to make a suprapubic cut into the abdomen. I could not, nor could those with me, understand why the bladder should be so high above the pelvis, and yet contain no urine. I explained to the mother (an Italian) the very desperate condition of her son, and, although he was sinking, determined to do what I could to relieve him. A very small quantity of ether sufficed to completely anæsthetize him, and I rapidly incised the bladder, which was empty, very much thickened, and very small. Upon introducing my finger into it, I found the roughened surface to cover up something extremely hard, and upon separating the tissue with my nail came upon a calculus situated in the prostate gland, occupying its entire area, and effectually closing the mouth of the urethra. It was with a great deal of difficulty that this stone could be dislodged, and it was only when one of my assistants introduced his finger into the rectum and forced up the stone that I could turn it out. The boy died in about an hour after the operation, and a post-mortem examination revealed an empty bladder, abscesses in both kidneys, a large quantity of pus in the pelvis of the right one, and an immense abscess, containing nearly a quart of matter, extending from the lower margin of the right kidney to the fundus of the bladder. The adhesions to the surrounding intestines and to the upper portion of the bladder were very numerous and dense, and thus raised that viscus out of the pelvis. I have not had this case inserted in the tables, for several reasons. First, because the operation was *not* undertaken as a suprapubic lithotomy, but to relieve a supposed extravasation, or as an entirely explorative one; second, because all the tables constituting the second chapter were then completed by Dr. Rankin, and ready for the printers; and, third, because of the bad condition of the boy for any operation whatsoever. The lesson, however, that it has taught me in the field of hypogastric section for stone, is this: that in children it is the most readily performed of any other operations of lithotomy. The time consumed in the performance of the operation was about four and a half minutes, the instruments, a small sound, a pair of forceps, and a curved bistoury.

Case V.—The following very interesting case occurred in the practice of my friend Dr. Doughty. I was present and assisted at both the operations.

M. O. D., a gentleman thirty-nine years old, had been troubled from early childhood with difficult and painful micturition. When about twelve years of age he had an attack of kidney colic, which was followed by cystitis, from which he suffered for the following four months, passing large quantities of pus, but no blood. The cystitis and general debility were so severe that his life was despaired of. He, however, rallied and regained good health, but the painful micturition continued to annoy him. With this exception, his health was good up to about twelve years ago, when he began to have frequently recurring attacks of chills, followed by fever and sweats, which were called malaria.

The difficulty in micturition and the so-called malarial chills becoming more severe, he was examined on May 30th, 1879, by his physician for stone and stricture, but neither was found. For the next four months he had urethral fever, intense pain on making water, and general debility. A considerable portion of this time he was confined to his bed.

In the early part of July, 1879, Dr. F. E. Doughty was called to take charge of the case. Although there were many of the symptoms of stone in the bladder, it did not seem advisable to make an examination at that time, on account of the fever, cystitis, and great debility of the patient, which condition was the result of the examination made May 30th. A change to a neighboring seaside resort, however, was recommended, where the patient remained one month, returning much improved in his general health, but the local symptoms remained about the same.

Dr. Doughty now determined to examine the bladder, and accordingly did so with the result of plainly detecting the presence of a large calculus. Lithotomy was accordingly proposed as the only means of relief, but the patient and his family would not consent to any cutting operation being performed. Dr. Doughty therefore decided to attempt litholapaxy, the patient insisting on having that operation performed. The urethra was prepared by dilatation, and sounds passed up to No. 16 English, the meatus having been cut.

On November 20th, 1879, ether having been administered, the crushing operation was attempted. There was no difficulty in clasping the stone, but on account of its immense size it was impossible to obtain sufficient purchase upon it to break it. Some small pieces were broken off, but the main portion remained intact. After two hours' fruitless endeavor, the operation was abandoned. The patient was put in bed and made as comfortable as possible. This was about 4 P.M., the operation having been commenced at about 2 o'clock. There was a great deal of nausea and vomiting from the ether. At 11.30 P.M., about 4 ounces of dark but not decidedly bloody urine were passed. There was only slight fever. Every three hours during the night he would pass 3 or 4 ounces of dark urine. On the morning after (November 21st), the temperature was $99\frac{3}{5}°$. Up to this time he had been unable to retain any nourishment; the vomiting now, however, ceased. He continued during the day, at intervals of about three hours, to pass his water, with intense pain, and with it a considerable number of broken bits of calculus were discharged. At 2.30 P.M., the temperature was 101°; in the evening, $101\frac{3}{5}°$, and the pulse 112. During the following night he continued to pass, with great pain, urine containing small bits of calculus. On November 22d, the second day after the operation, there was more calcareous debris discharged every time the bladder was emptied, and the pain on micturition was more severe than before. The temperature during the day was normal and the pulse 88. The general condition was about the same. There was some tenderness over the hypogastric region.

For the next three days the symptoms remained unchanged; every few hours he would urinate, with great suffering, passing dark-colored and now occasionally, bloody urine, with broken bits of calculus.

On November 25th, it was decided to perform suprapubic lithotomy, the patient now having consented to any measure likely to give him relief. Up to this time the most nutritious and easily digested food had been given, and at different intervals, arsenic and brandy, with an occasional hypodermic injection of Magendie (12 in all).

The operation was performed after the following manner: The patient, after being thoroughly anæsthetized, was placed on the table and the bladder injected with about 12 ounces of water carbolized. The incision was made in the linea alba, and the bladder easily reached. It was then secured by means of a loop of catgut, and held in position. The bladder was then punctured, from within outward, by means of the "*sonde-à-dard*," just above the pubes, and with the knife an incision was made upward and downward to the desired extent. The finger was now passed into the bladder, and immediately came in contact with a large calculus.

Forceps were then introduced, and after considerable difficulty, including an extension of the incision to the utmost limits admissible, a calculus of uric acid, weighing three (3) ounces and one hundred and fifty (150) grains, was extracted. The diameters of the stone were 2¾ inches × 2 inches × 1¾ inches. Several good-sized pieces, the result of the previous operation, were also removed; which with the debris washed out at first sitting, plus that obtained by filtering the urine voided between the operations, gave 96 grains additional, making in all a calculus weighing three ounces and two hundred and forty-eight grains.

The bladder was now washed, and the edges brought together by means of interrupted sutures of catgut. The external wound was closed by silver sutures. A drainage-tube was introduced at the bottom of the wound, and a soft rubber catheter tied into the bladder, via the urethra.

There was no nausea or vomiting after this second operation, whereas these symptoms had been very troublesome in the first. At 7 P.M., there were two ounces of not very bloody urine in the bottle, and about three ounces on a towel. By midnight half a gill more had collected, quite clear. He was feverish and complained of much pain   ℞. Aconite θ, followed by a hypodermic injection of fifteen minims of Magendie.

5.45 A.M., November 26th, temperature 100½°; gave eight minims of Magendie.

8 A.M., six ounces of clear urine in the bottle.

10 A.M., has considerable pain and is much distended with wind, which he

is unable to expel. Temperature 100½°, pulse 128. Clear urine continues to collect. Gave eight minims more of Magendie solution.

3 P.M., is suffering severely again from wind. Gave Magendie again, same dose as before.

5.30 P.M., temperature 98½°, pulse 128.

10 P.M., dressed wound; pulse 116, temperature 98½°. ℞. Chin.θ.

November 27th, 1.30 A.M., temperature 98½°. Starts suddenly every fifteen or twenty minutes while asleep; knees are quite cold. There are about three ounces of urine in the bottle. ℞. Belladonnaθ, followed at 3.15 A.M. by seven minims of Magendie's solution, after which he slept for three-quarters of an hour without any spasms.

4.30 A.M., gave some flaxseed tea. 6.30, started out of his sleep with a spasm. Dressed the wound at this hour. 10.45 A.M., pulse 129, temperature 100°.

1.30 P.M., dressed wound, and removed suspensory ligature. Pulse 104, temperature 98°.

5.15 P.M., complains of feeling bad all over; pulse good; is quite chilly and cold. Gave brandy, egg and milk.

5.30 P.M., ℞. Ars., 3ˣ, Bell.θ.

8.30 P.M., dressed wound, catheter a little coated; pulse 100, temperature 98°.

November 28th, continues in about the same condition. Beef tea and milk are given at short intervals. The temperature and pulse keep about 100, and 98½° respectively. The wound looks healthy, and clear urine collects in the bottle every two or three hours.

November 29th, 1 P.M., no urine has passed through the catheter since 7 A.M. Removed it, and found it plugged; cleaned and reintroduced it. Pulse 100, temperature 98⅞°. At 3 P.M., there was a return of the spasms, for which Bell.θ. was given hourly, with relief.

November 30th, improving a little. During the morning there were a few spasmodic twitchings, which Bell.θ again relieved.

11 A.M., is sleepless and uneasy. ℞. Magendie solution, ♏12.

6 P.M., pulse 112, temperature 100½°; suffers considerable pain; has had Verat. vir.θ for the last two hours.

8 P.M., is less feverish; pulse 106. ℞. Chinaθ, alt. ars. 3ˣ. Dressed the wound at this hour and removed the catheter for cleansing; urine runs through the catheter freely.

December 1st, urine comes out almost entirely by the wound; very little of it collecting in the bottle from the catheter; rearranged the dressings, catheter, and tube; feels to-day quite well excepting a slight chilliness; the night previous there was a little sweating. Pulse 100, temperature 99½°. ℞. Ignat.θ.

In the evening gave a free injection into the bowels of soap and oil; urine by catheter.

December 2d, urine free; enema repeated; dressed wound as usual.

December 3d, removed one suture; wound not completely united; removed catheter.

December 4th, 2 A.M., slept well up to this hour; free discharge from the tube; sometimes the tube will not carry anything off, while on the other hand, there will be a free discharge from it; gave seven minims of Magendie's solution.

December 5th, has a little fever to-day; temperature 100°. R. Aconite θ. Introduced new drainage-tube with shield, which seems to be very effectual in preventing the urine overflowing.

December 8, 8 A.M., temperature 99⅔°, pulse 100, condition good; slept well last night; at 7 P.M., was troubled with spasmodic contractions of the muscles of the groins and rectum. R. Ignat. θ alt. ars., followed by eleven minims of Magendie's solution.

December 9th, has had more spasms, very severe; gave fifteen minims of Magendie. In the evening, fourteen minims more of Magendie; pulse 100, and temperature 101°.

December 10th, 1.30 A.M., is very restless and sleepless. R. Magendie*, followed by Hyos. θ. 3 P.M. R. Pod. 1*, gr. xv, and then Moschus every two hours. At 10 P.M. R. Chloral hyd., gr. xv, and at 12 o'clock, Chloral hyd., gr. v; 1.45 A.M. R. Chloral hyd., gr. iv.

December 11th, 6.30, has had a free evacuation of the bowels, and has slept considerably.

December 12th, to-day the wound is looking nicely and is gradually healing.

The records of the patient's condition for the next ten days show a gradual improvement; enough Morph. sulph. was given to cause sleep. The bladder was washed out as often as occasion required. The pulse remained for some time 120, but fell to normal point on the return of strength.

After the application of the shield over the wound, no difficulty was experienced, it completely conveying all the urine into the receiver.

A small fistula remained for some weeks, but finally closed under the application of a probe coated with nitrate of silver.

I here insert the cases of Mr. Fowler and Mr. Hutchinson as being recent and interesting cases of lithotomy, where the suprapubic operation was resorted to in consequence of the size of the stone.

Mr. R. S. Fowler* reports the case of a boy, aged 16, who was admitted as a patient into the Royal United Hospital, on November 9th, 1877, suffering

---

* British Medical Journal, September 7th, 1878.

PLATE VI. (page 82)

Case V.—M.O.D. age 39. Merchant. The lines for the 21st and 22nd of December, indicate pulse and Temperature after ineffectual litholapaxy. Supra-pubic lithotomy was performed on the 25th of December, and after the 9th of that month, the progress of the case was regular and unnecessary to report.

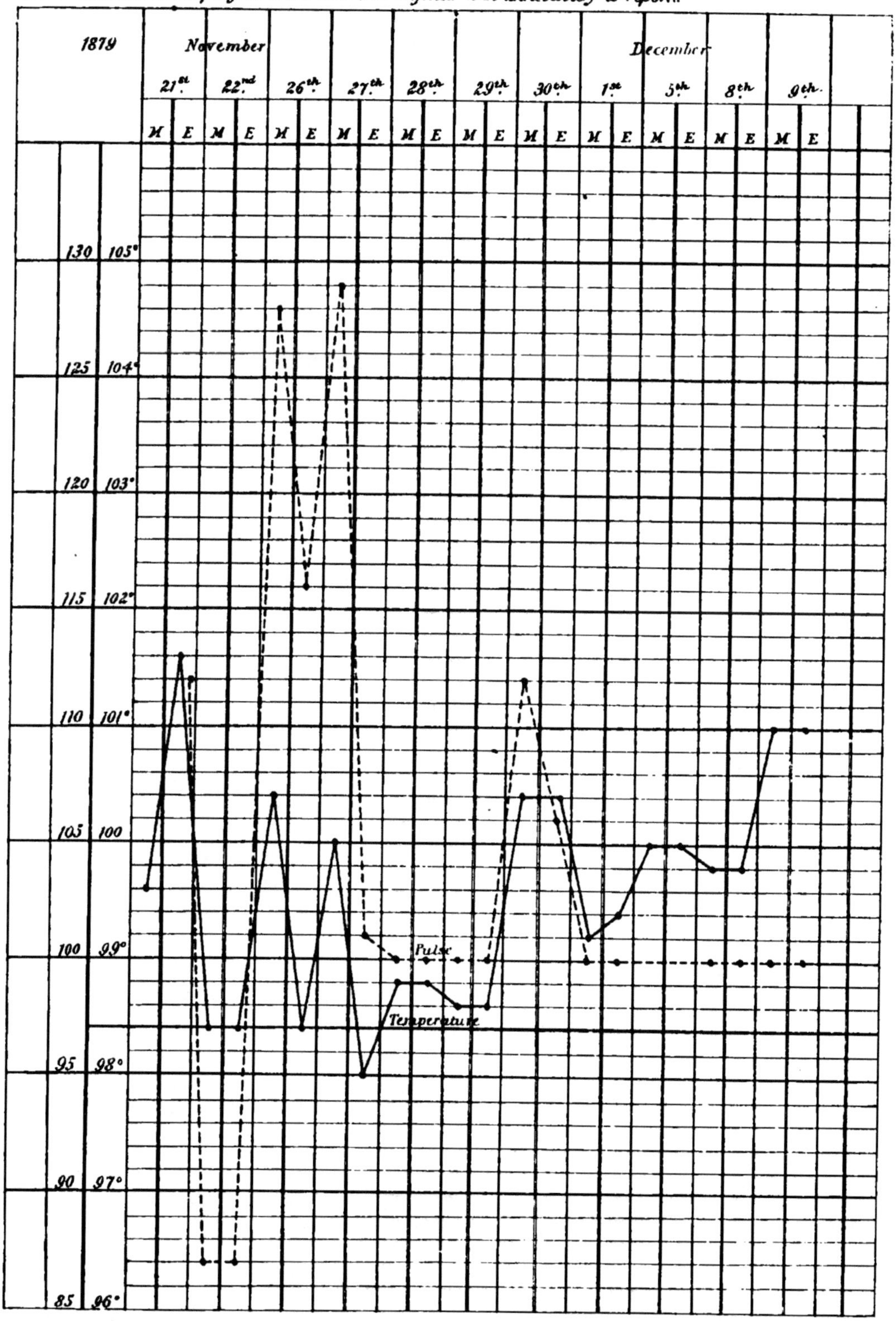

1879
November
December
21st
22nd
26th
27th
28th
29th
30th
1st
5th
8th
9th
M E M E M E M E M E M E M E M E M E M E M E
130 105°
125 104°
120 103°
115 102°
110 101°
105 100
100 99°
95 98°
90 97°
85 96°
Pulse
Temperature

from all the symptoms of calculus in the bladder. On November 14th, Mr. Fowler operated by the lateral section, but was unable from the great size of the stone to extract it. Attempts at crushing being unsuccessful, it was decided to proceed to hypogastric lithotomy; the stone was held against the anterior wall of the bladder, while Mr. Fowler cut down upon it, and making a crucial incision, readily extracted it. The patient did very well. The wound above the pubes rapidly healed, but the perineal opening gave some annoyance for several months, but eventually was closed by a plastic operation. "The calculus, oxalate of lime, was nearly circular, one inch and a half in diameter, covered with mulberry excrescences, and weighed two ounces. The boy is now in good health, and engaged in heavy work as an errand boy."*

Mr. Hutchinson's Case.

"At a late meeting of the Clinical Society of London (*Medical Times and Gazette*, October 19th, 1878), Mr. Jonathan Hutchinson read notes of this case, which was that of a man, aged about twenty-six, who had suffered from symptoms of stone for about six months. When admitted into the hospital his condition was urgent, the bladder being exceedingly irritable, and the urine containing pus and blood. He was considerably emaciated. There was no difficulty in recognizing that the stone was a very large one, and careful consideration was given to the question of the best means of extracting it. It was finally decided to prefer the suprapubic method. No difficulty was encountered in the operation; the bladder was easily reached; and, the wound having been adequately enlarged, the stone was seized in the largest pair of forceps. Its size necessitated a little delay in extraction to allow the soft parts to yield. After its removal an india-rubber tube was passed through the urethra and retained in the bladder. It was hoped by this means to drain away the urine without any wetting of the bed. The fundus of the bladder was found much thickened and quite rigid by calcareous deposit. For the first week after the operation the man did exceedingly well; he then began to lose flesh, and subsequently had repeated rigors. The urine contained pus, and was constantly ammoniacal. Although great attention was given to the bladder, it was found impossible to keep it empty and avoid overflow on the edges of the wound. The patient died of pyæmia about five weeks after the operation. At the necropsy the bladder was found very much thickened by inflammation, and its mucous membrane ulcerated and coated with concretion. The kidneys contained abscesses, and there were small pyæmic deposits in the liver and lungs. The calculus removed was very hard and heavy, of lithic acid, weighing nearly six ounces

* Monthly Abstract of Medical Sciences, December, 1878.

and a half, and measuring nine inches in circumference at the greatest, and six at the least width. Mr. Hutchinson showed also the cast of a calculus, of almost exactly the same size and weight as his own, which had been removed at the London Hospital, by the late Mr. John Adams, about ten years ago. In this instance, the unusual size of the stone was unexpected, and the ordinary lateral operation was adopted. The patient, who was a healthy young man, recovered well."

Professor Trendelenberg has also reported a successful case of suprapubic lithotomy.* The patient was a child two years old. The stone, readily felt through the rectum, was pushed up by the finger in the anus, and the incision made directly over it. The after-treatment consisted in leaving the wound free, and turning the patient on the belly,—the position recommended by this surgeon.

* London Medical Record, February 16th, 1877.

CHAPTER V.

METHOD OF PERFORMING EPICYSTOTOMY.

In looking over the many directions for the performance of suprapubic lith-otomy, I must say that I think a good deal of stress has been laid on unimportant steps of the operation. To my mind it makes but little difference whether the incision be made with a bistoury or scalpel, whether it goes from above downward, or below upward, whether the bladder be held up with a tenaculum, or a hooked finger, or a loop of catgut, provided it *be* held up. An operating surgeon will have his favorite instruments, which, in his hands, have been best

Fig. 1.

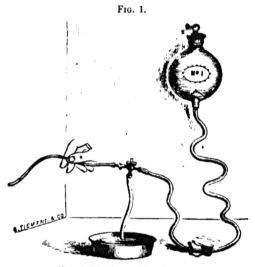

Keyes's Bladder-washing Apparatus.

adapted for making the appropriate incisions. Several days before the operation, if the urine has been putrid, or there has been atony of the bladder, that viscus should be washed out carefully with a saturated aqueous solution of the biborate of soda, and the best apparatus for the purpose is that of Dr. Keyes, as represented in Fig. 1. To the extremity of the tube of a fountain syringe, No. 1, is attached a nickel-plated "two way" stopcock. On one of the "ways," the catheter, metallic or flexible, is attached; to the other "way," a bit of india-rubber tubing leading off into a basin. The ordinary stopcock belonging to the syringe is also of service in regulating the flow. The bag is filled with the saturated borax solution, and the stopcock of the instrument turned in a line with the catheter; this allows the bladder to gradually fill. So soon as the patient desires to evacuate the bladder, the stopcock is turned in the opposite direction and the water flows out.

Whether the bladder is injected before the operation is of undoubted importance. In my opinion it should be distended as much as possible to elevate the peritonæum. The sonde-à-dard is also not an essential; a catheter or ordinary sound will mark the point where the bladder incision should terminate if begun at the pelvis, or where it should be begun if it terminates at the pubes. It, however, gives a sure guide to a free, bold, and smooth incision into the bladder, and should, I think, therefore be used if practicable. Besides this, in the modification of it which I have devised, it prevents the frequent passage of instruments through the urethra, which in some cases is not desirable.

Fig. 2.

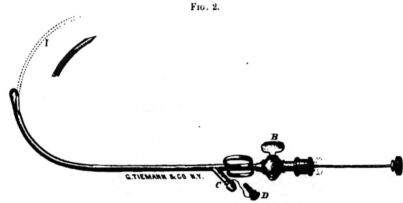

The Author's modification of the Sonde-à-dard.

Every instrument must be "listered," every particle of the bedclothing, the clothing, atmosphere, and apparatus, should be prepared with great care; then,

1. Place the patient in a comfortable position supine, on a table of proper height, and administer the anæsthetic.

2. Introduce the sonde-à-dard, Fig. 2, without the stilette, and inject the bladder, with stopcock *B* open, with a solution of Calendula 1–100, at a temperature of 100°. So soon as the slightest resistance to the passage of liquid is observed, draw the plug from the mouth of the flange *C,* and, as the water passes out, inject more until the bladder is thoroughly cleaned.

3. Insert the plug *D* firmly into its place, and inject the bladder with as much as it will hold, and, having done this, turn the stopcock to retain the water.

It will be seen by this, that the sonde may be used not only as a searcher for the stone, but for injecting and washing out the bladder, and that if it be made the proper size, equal to a No. 16 English bougie, there will little, if any, water escape by its side. By using one instrument a great advantage is gained, especially in cases of sensitive urethræ, where the frequent introduction and withdrawal of tubes may very greatly complicate the case.

The instrument used to inject is the ordinary rubber 12-ounce syringe, Fig. 3, also fitted with a stopcock.

4. The surgeon then with a scalpel makes an incision from a point about two inches and a half above the pubic symphysis in the line of the linea alba, down to the top of the pubis, and about *half an inch over the top of the pubic arch*, almost to the root of the penis.

This extension of incision is of import, for it gives room to manipulate instruments, and in persons in whom there is much adipose tissue, this latter part of the cut assists materially in widening the mouth of the pit.

While making this cut, by holding a small sponge with the middle, ring and little finger (after the manner in which an apothecary holds the cork of a vial which he is decanting into another bottle), and rendering the integument tense with the thumb and finger of the same hand, the surgeon may do his own sponging, and keep the cut clean as he goes through the tissues.

5. When the linea alba is reached, the parts are examined to see if there be any bleeding points; if there be, the vessels may be twisted, or small catch-forceps, as first recommended by Spencer Wells, may be applied, or Vidal's forceps may be employed. The lips of the wound may then be more widely separated by pushing them apart with the fingers.

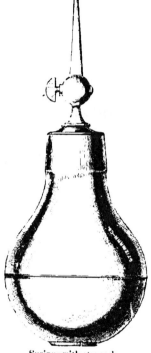

Fig. 3.

Syringe with stopcock.

6. The tendinous expansion must then be snipped above the pubes, a director inserted, and the abdomen opened from below upward for at least two inches. I generally do this with the scissors, although a knife with a probe point or a sharp-pointed curved bistoury will do as well. This brings the fat, which is usually found about the fundus of the bladder, in view, and as in my first case it gave me much perplexity, on account of its quantity, it is well to remember that it is often found of considerable thickness. If the cut is extended higher towards the umbilicus, the peritonæum is brought into view, but as a rule, this is not necessary.

7. At this stage of the operation the handle of the sonde-à-dard must gradually be depressed between the legs of the patient to bring its beak at the

fundus of the bladder, just below the point of attachment of the peritonæum; thus the surgeon has a guide to this most important point in the anatomy of the operation.

8. The assistant holding the instrument as above, the surgeon takes a round curved needle, threaded with strong, carbolized catgut, passes it through the bladder-wall, draws it through, ties a knot in the catgut, making a loop of about an inch and a half, cuts off the needle and places the loop over the bent finger of an assistant. Or fenestrated catch-forceps may be used.

9. The stopcock (B) of the sonde is then turned, and a good portion of the fluid allowed to run off. This is done to prevent any water escaping into the cavity of the abdomen, as the stilette is passed through the bladder.

10. The stilette (C) is then pushed into the canula and passed directly through the bladder. *Vide* Plate VII, Fig. 1.

11. The sharp point of a pair of scissors or the point of a curved bistoury, or the curved probe-pointed aponeurotome, as seen in the cut, Fig. 4 (I pre-

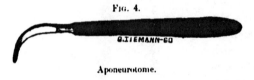

FIG. 4.

G.TIEMANN-CO

Aponeurotome.

fer the former) is introduced into the groove of the stilette, and the incision enlarged sufficiently to get a fair opening into the bladder. *Vide* Plate VII, Fig. 2. The stilette is then withdrawn into the sonde, which also is entirely removed from the bladder, it being kept well up by the loop of gut on the finger of an assistant.

12. The finger is then gently introduced into the bladder, and the stone or stones are at once perceived, and in the majority of instances the fingers are the instruments with which to remove the calculi. When, however, the concretions are large or the patient very fat, as in my first case, forceps must be employed and used with the utmost gentleness, until the calculus is grasped and removed. *Vide* Plate VIII, Fig. 1.

13. Search must then be made to be certain that the bladder is entirely free from all stones, and then the bladder-wound must be sewn up.

14. In sewing up the bladder, whether indeed it should be sewn or not, has been a matter of discussion. Great care should be used, and fine needles threaded with fine catgut employed. In my own cases and in that of Dr. Doughty, in every instance, the bladder-wound was closed with carbolized sutures of catgut. To do this effectually, a fine piece of the gut should be threaded upon a small-sized curved needle, and a small knot tied at the end; beginning at the top of the wound, just below the point of suspension of the bladder by the loop of catgut already mentioned, a glover's or continued suture should be carried the whole length of the wound, a reverse stitch then taken and the needle cut away.

PLATE VII.

Fig. 1

H
B
K
B
C
A
J
I
G
F
E
D

Fig. 2

k
C
G
H
A
F
E
D
I

H. Faber. ft.

G. Moras. lith. Phila.

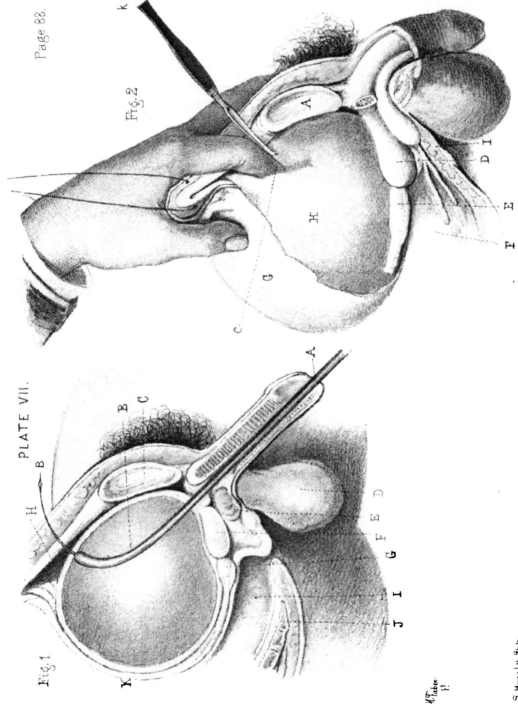

PLATE VII.

Fig. 1.—Section of Pelvis showing Action of the Sonde-λ-Dard.

A. Meatus urinarius external.

B. Sonde-à-dard within the bladder, with the bulb against the anterior wall, and the stilette B¹ carried over the pubis and through the abdominal wall.

C. Symphysis pubis.

D. Scrotum.

E. Urethral bulb.

F. Prostate gland.

G. Vesicula seminalis.

H. Triangular space on anterior face of the fundus of bladder uncovered by the peritoneum.

I. Rectum.

J. Coccyx.

K. Posterior wall of bladder covered by peritoneum.

Fig. 2.—Showing Method of Incising Bladder.

A. Symphysis pubis.

B. Loop holding bladder.

C. Bladder wall incised, with finger dilating the incision to search for stone.

D. Prostate gland.

E. Vesicula seminalis.

F. Rectum.

G. Posterior wall of bladder covered by peritoneum.

H. Bladder.

I. Anus.

K. Curved bistoury in position.

Günther does not apply any stitches whatsoever, but Starr sews the walls of the abdomen and the bladder-wound with a peculiar stitch, which includes both the bladder and the walls of the abdomen. He says of it: "I passed a silver suture down through the wall of the abdomen into the cavity of the bladder, included a part of this and brought the wire back through the bladder and abdominal wall on the same side, then I carried it across the incision, passed it down through the abdominal wall and bladder on this side, included a segment here, and brought it out as before, and just opposite where it had first entered the tissues. Now when the ends of the suture were drawn upon, the sides of the wound were approximated, but the edges of the incision in the bladder were inverted and their outer surfaces brought into contact, while the mucous surfaces were turned inward, thus promoting union."*

15. After the bladder-wound has been sewn (that is, if it be not included with the abdominal walls after the manner of Dr. Starr), a sponge-holder containing antiseptic absorbent cotton must be gently pressed within the wound, to remove all the clots, moisture, etc., that may have accumulated, but sufficient force must not be used to separate any of the paravesical connective tissue.

Fig. 5.

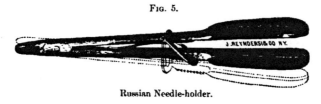

Russian Needle-holder.

16. The loop of catgut must then be drawn to the top of the wound, where, however, it generally remains, and held there while the tegumentary cut is closed.

In my last case, instead of using the catgut loop, I held up the bladder with a pair of forceps with a spring-catch on the handles and broad fenestrated blades.

17. In sewing the abdomen-wound, either one of two methods will be found serviceable. A large-sized round needle should be threaded with a waxed silk thread, which should be cut to leave ends about four inches long; these ends should be sewn together with fine thread, or be spliced together to make a loop. This method, which I have used for many years, is better than tying the half knot. The loop must then again be waxed; upon this the silver wire No. 26 must be bent, and squeezed together with a pair of forceps. By this means the extreme flexibility of the silk allows the needle to be inserted and withdrawn through the abdominal walls without kinking the wire. I may say here, that the best of all needle-holders, especially where the tissues are thick, is that known as the Russian, Fig. 5.

* American Journal of the Medical Sciences, July, 1877, p. 113.

12

The needle is introduced about half an inch from the margin of the cut at the upper angle of the wound, passed through the entire thickness of the abdominal wall, and drawn through; again it is grasped by the needle-holder, inserted in the opposite side under the tissues, and brought out at the integument at a point opposite to where it has been entered on the other margin of the cut. The silver wire is then drawn gently through and cut off, to leave about an inch and a half projecting from each side of the incision. These two ends are immediately taken in charge by an assistant, who turns them over on the abdomen towards the head of the patient. A second suture is introduced in like manner about a quarter of an inch from the first, and so on; the lips of the wound are brought in close proximity, leaving, however, about half an inch at the lower angle for the admission of the drainage-tube.

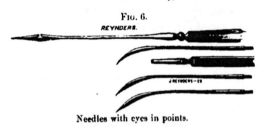

Fig. 6.
REYNDERS.

Needles with eyes in points.

The second method for the introduction of the wires, is to take a needle, with an eye in its point, Fig. 6, thread it with a piece of waxed silk about four inches long, introduce it from within outward, and when the eye with the thread in it appears at the integument, draw it (the thread) forward with a small tenaculum, until the loop is sufficiently large to hook upon it the wire, which is then bent over the thread. The needle is then withdrawn, the operator taking care to hold in his grasp, with the handle of the instrument, the distal extremity of the silk. The operation is repeated in a similar manner on the opposite side. As each wire is introduced, the assistant turns the ends upward, as in the first instance, and holds them out of the way until a sufficient number are introduced.

18. Then, before the parts are approximated, the spray apparatus is brought to bear over the entire surface, and again the sponge-holder, charged with fresh antiseptic cotton, is carefully used to remove any blood that may have oozed from the needle-puncture.

19. A small-sized glass drainage-tube, having a flange, to which is attached a piece of new india-rubber tubing, is inserted into the lower angle of the wound, and then the wires are twisted with the usual instrument. A new cork must be placed in the drainage-tube, and the india-rubber tube carried over the thigh of the patient into a vessel, containing carbolized water, on the floor, or upon a stool by the edge of the bed. A narrow strip of plaster must then be laid along one side of the wound, and the ends of the wires, bent over the point of a tenaculum, turned down. Over the whole wound, a good covering of marine lint should be placed, and secured by means of carbolized india-rubber plaster.

20. The loop of catgut must then be lowered a little, and secured by placing

PLATE VIII.

Page 9.

Fig. 2

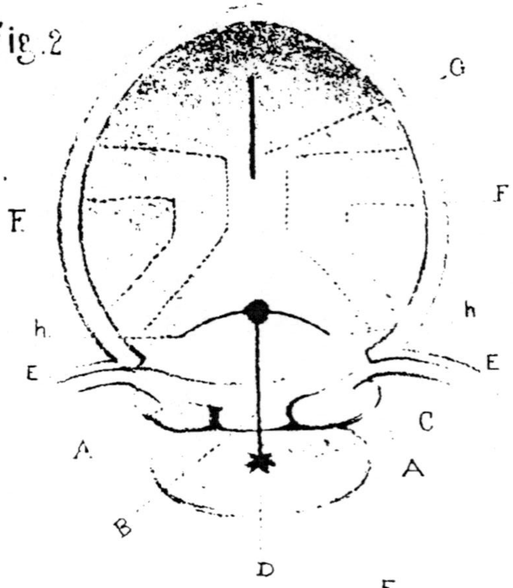
G
F
F
h
h
E
E
C
A
A
B
D

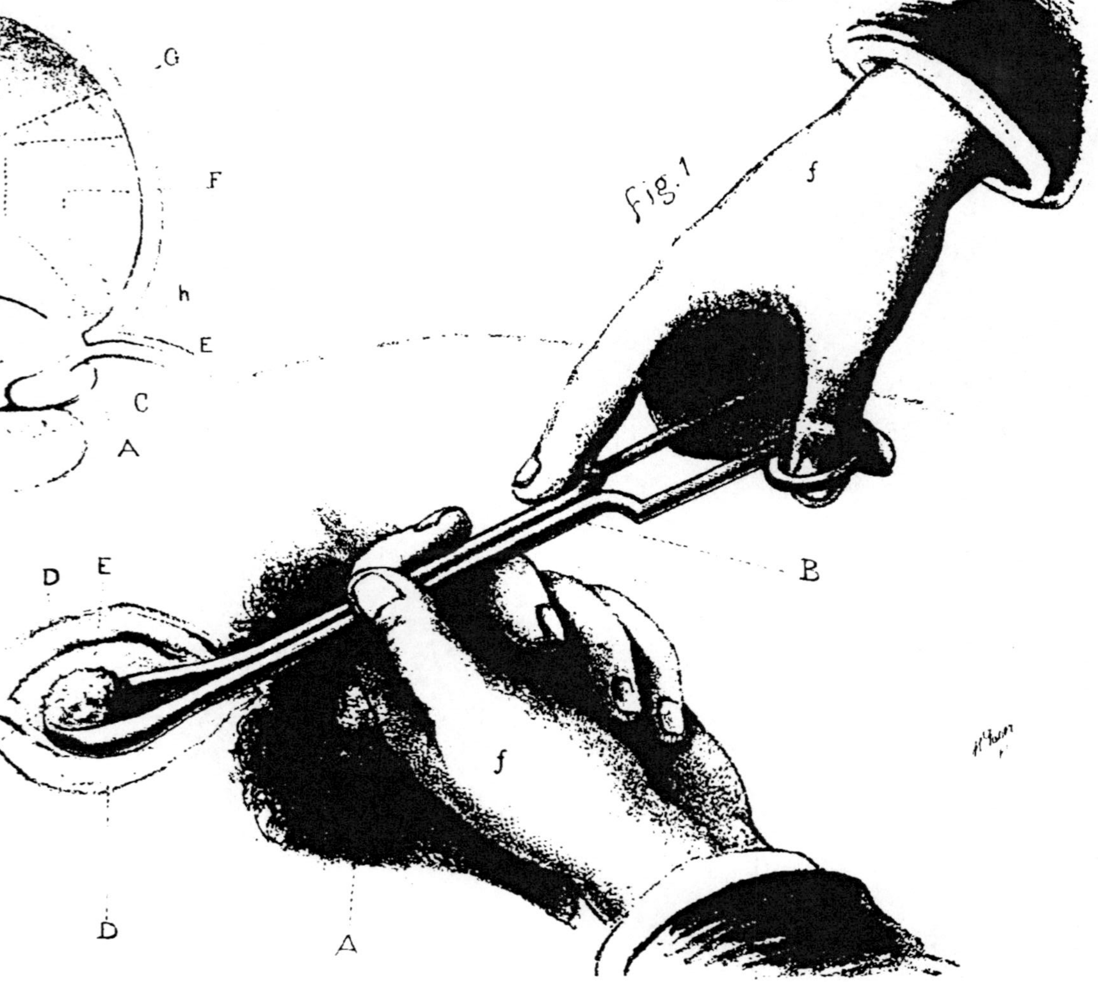
Fig. 1
f
f
B
D
E
C
D
A

J. Moras lith Phila

PLATE VIII.

FIG. 1.—REMOVAL OF STONE WITH FORCEPS THROUGH THE ABDOMINAL INCISION.

A. Symphysis pubis.

B. Forceps closed upon the stone.

C. Calculus in jaws of forceps.

D. Integumental cut.

E. Bladder wall.

F. Position of the hands of operator.

FIG. 2.—INTERNAL ASPECT OF BLADDER WITH REMOVAL OF THE POSTERIOR WALL, SHOWING THE VARIED INCISIONS FOR LITHOTOMY. THE DOTTED LINES REP-RESENT THE SYMPHYSIS PUBIS AND ANTERIOR CUL-DE-SAC OF BLADDER.

AA. Vesiculæ seminales.

B. Antero-posterior line from neck of bladder to rectum, showing bladder wound in recto-vesical lithotomy.

C. Rectum.

D. Anus.

EE. Vasa-deferentia and ureters.

FF. Bladder wall.

G. Vertical incision for suprapubic lithotomy.

HH. Semilunar incision, with anterior convexity made in the bas-fond of bladder in bi-lateral method; one side of this line marks the entrance to the bladder in the lateral operation.

a bit of bougie through the loop transversely over the incision, and holding the bougie in the abdomen by adhesive strips. I use this as an additional preventive for extravasation; the idea being to keep the bladder-walls somewhat apart, and thus making a somewhat deeper trough for the accumulation of the urine.

Whether this has accomplished its purpose, I cannot say, for I have always been very careful to keep the bladder empty by the presence of the catheter, or its frequent application. Dr. Doughty has invented a most ingenious and, in his hands, a most satisfactory apparatus to prevent excoriation from overflowing urine, which ought to be used as soon as the urine shows itself through the abdominal wall. It consists (Fig. 7) of a glass bell similar to a nipple-shield, which, for convenience of illustration, we divide as follows: A, bell; B, flange; C, rest. At the junction of A and B, is an aperture for the passage of the drainage-tube. This must fit snugly, and must be of sufficient length to pass from a bottle, between the thighs, over the scrotum, by the side of the penis, through the aperture in the bell, and well into the wound. The end of the drainage-tube in the bottle must be lower than the bladder, that it may act as a siphon. The tube must have openings at intervals in all that part of it within the wound, and one, on its upper side, within the bell, just where it has passed the aperture. Let the pubes be shaved, the drainage-tube be introduced, and the wound, unless there has been primary union, be brought together with adhesive strips (as applied to an ordinary indolent ulcer), leaving the lower inch of it exposed. In applying the instrument, let the centre of the bell correspond with the lower extremity of the incision, to admit of an easy introduction of the tube into the wound. To secure it in its place, let a strip of adhesive plaster, six inches in length by one in width, with a semicircular piece cut from one edge in the middle to receive the bell, be applied across the wound and over the flange. Next, let a

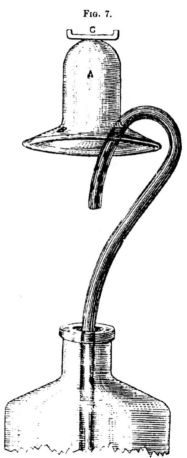

FIG. 7.

Doughty's apparatus to prevent excoriation from overflowing urine.

piece of roller bandage be passed under the patient, and the ends brought up over the thighs just above the great trochanters, leaving the space across the abdomen for the attachment (by pinning or sewing) of a piece of elastic, ¼ to ¾ of an inch in width, and without tension. Raise the elastic from its centre to the rest C. The roller bandage and the elastic being properly adjusted, no urine can escape on the person, nor can any suffering be experienced by the patient. Therefore, the utmost skill and precision in the application of the apparatus is indispensable to the desired result. For, *unless the pubes be equally impressed by the entire flange, and so that no pain result to the patient from too severe pressure*, the application is a failure. The reasons and the remedies are both obvious. If the failure is due to the roller bandage (causing tipping of the bell, and so unequal pressure of the flange), it must be newly adjusted by removing it, either a trifle higher or lower; if it is due to the elastic, its tension must be increased or diminished. Stoppage of the tube external to the bell will be readily detected by the rising of the urine within it (the bell), and can be relieved by aspiration, by means of a small penis syringe. If the obstruction is in the part within the wound, the whole apparatus must be removed, for reasons readily appreciated.

It is a question with some surgeons regarding drainage. Dr. Stimson says that Dr. Keyes recommended drainage per rectum ; others draw off the water every few hours, as recommended by Dulles. I have seen most excellent results from fixing a Nélaton flexible catheter in the bladder, only removing it sufficiently often to cleanse it, recollecting that so soon as its bladder-end shows a tendency to become rough, a new one must be substituted for the old one.

21. The position the patient assumes makes but little difference, but for the first few days the recumbent one is that most desired by the patient, because it is the most comfortable. As for renewal of the old practice of turning the patient on the face, as lately practiced by Trendelenberg, I should think it both undesirable and tiresome, and above all, the position would be likely to force the urine from the wound, simply by attraction of gravitation, one of the circumstances which is of all the most to be deprecated in the after-treatment of the operation.

AFTER-TREATMENT.

There can be no doubt that the chief danger in " the high operation " for stone consists in the liability to urinary infiltration, and, perhaps, phlegmonous inflammation of the paravesical tissues. The wounding of the peritonæum, I should think, need never occur, excepting in cases in which the enormous size of a calculus necessitated a corresponding wound in the bladder, and in such, indeed, it would be preferable to crush the stone and remove it by fragments; that is, if the stone can be broken, which may be found difficult in some cases.

I am of opinion that the evil results of urinary extravasation can be very much reduced by the method I have lately practiced. The next morning after the operation the patient should be dressed as follows : All the bandages should be removed and the parts carefully washed and dried ; then a coating of flexible collodion should be placed over the wound and around it, for the distance of three or four inches on each side, and down on the inside of the thighs. The drainage-tube should then be removed ; if glass, it must be cleansed and allowed to lie in a solution of carbolic acid 1–60 until it is wanted ; if india-rubber, it is to be burned and a new one employed. A flexible Nélaton catheter, with a countersunk eye, is then to be attached to the tube of a fountain-syringe, and carbolized water 1–100, at a temperature of 100°, allowed to run into the wound; this should be continued until a quart of the solution has been so used. Then the dresser, taking his probe, wraps the end of it with borated cotton, introduces it to the depth of the incision, and wipes out the wound; he then removes the cotton, reapplies another piece, uses it in like manner, and so on continues until the whole cavity is dry. This may take half an hour or even more. The catheter also is removed from the bladder, washed and carbolized, and is ready for readjustment.

The surface of the abdomen must then be covered with a large wad of borated absorbent cotton, and a muslin binder applied over it, and securely fastened with safety-pins. The catheter for the first few days must be perma- nently retained in the bladder, which is best accomplished as follows : Take six or eight hooks, such as are used in fastening ladies' dresses (hooks and eyes), secure three of them just below the glans penis, by wrapping around the organ a strap of india-rubber salicylated adhesive plaster, apply a corresponding number to the flexible catheter at a point about an inch from the meatus, after the catheter is inserted, and by slipping over both corresponding hooks a small india-rubber band, which from its elasticity will allow sufficient expansion of the penis, which sometimes has a tendency to erect, or at least enlarge, the instrument will be comfortably kept in position. After the first week, the per- manent use of the catheter should be dispensed with, and the urine drawn every two or three hours.

NOTE.—In concluding this monograph, the Author would state, that the greater portion of it (comprising most of the first, third and fourth chapters), was prepared in 1878–79, and constituted his Thesis for admission to the Medico-Chirurgical Society of New York.

Dr. Rankin's table, forming the second chapter, was constructed later, and also was accepted as his Thesis for membership to the same organization.

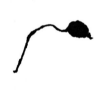

Lightning Source UK Ltd.
Milton Keynes UK
31 July 2010

157669UK00004B/32/P